Medical Innovations in Humanitarian Situations

The Work of Médecins Sans Frontières

Edited by Jean-Hervé Bradol and Claudine Vidal

Translated by Christopher Brasher, Nina Friedman, Philippa Bowe Smith, Karen Stokes, and Karen Tucker

Acknowledgements

We wish to thank: Kate Albertini *(N, E)*, Isabelle Baszanger *(S)*, Dounia Bitar *(D, E)*, Christopher Brasher *(D)*, Rony Brauman *(D)*, Marilyn Bonnet *(D, E)*, Laurence Bonte *(La)*, Vincent Brown *(D, E)*, Maurice Cassier *(S)*, Bérengère Cescau *(A)*, François Chapuis *(D)*, Francisco Diaz *(Lg)*, Ali Djibo *(D)*, Stéphane Doyon *(A)*, François Enten *(S)*, Florence Fermon *(N)*, Renée C. Fox *(S)*, Marc Gastellu-Etchegorry *(D, E)*, Rebecca Freeman Grais *(E)*, Philippe Guérin *(D, E)*, Jean-Paul Guthmann *(E)*, Annick Hamel *(N)*, Geza Harczi *(N)*, Myriam Henkens *(D)*, Northan Hurtado *(D)*, Guy Jacquier *(E)*, Unni Karanakura *(D)*, Dominique Legros *(D, E)*, Alain Moren *(D, E)*, Marylin Mulemba *(N)*, Christophe Paquet *(D, E)*, Patrice Piola *(D, E)*, Gerardo Priotto *(D, E)*, Bernard Pécoul *(D, E)*, Michel Rey *(D)*, Jean Rigal *(D)*, Malika Saim *(N)*, Fatouma Sidikou *(D)*, Mike Toole *(D, E)*, Michel Van Herp *(D, E)*, Brigitte Vasset *(D)*, Rony Waldman *(D, E)*, Fabrice Weissman *(P)*.

We thank them for their time, advice, participation in text-review sessions, availability for interviews on MSF's medical practices, as well as many other forms of assistance.

Thanks to them, the editors never felt alone.

(A) administrator, (E) epidemiologist, (N) nurse, (La) laboratory technician, (Lg) logistician, (D) doctor, (P) political scientist, (S) sociologist

Contributors

Dr. Suna Balkan, *medical department, MSF, Paris.*

Dr. Emmanuel Baron, *epidemiologist, Epicentre.*

Dr. Jean-Hervé Bradol, *Centre de réflexion sur l'action et les savoirs humanitaires (Crash), Fondation Médecins Sans Frontières.*

Dr. Jean-François Corty, *Centre de réflexion sur l'action et les savoirs humanitaires (Crash), Fondation Médecins Sans Frontières.*

Dr. Eugénie d'Alessandro, *Centre de réflexion sur l'action et les savoirs humanitaires (Crash), Fondation Médecins Sans Frontières.*

Dr. Isabelle Defourny, *department of operations, MSF, Paris.*

Nicolas Dodier, *sociologist, Groupe de sociologie politique et morale, Ecole des hautes études en sciences sociales.*

Marc Le Pape, *sociologist, Centre d'Études africaines, Ecole des hautes études en sciences sociales.*

Jacques Pinel, *pharmacist, medical department, MSF, Paris.*

Dr. Elisabeth Szumilin, *medical department, MSF, Paris.*

Claudine Vidal, *sociologist, Groupe de sociologie politique et morale, Ecole des hautes études en sciences sociales.*

Contents

Medical Innovations in Humanitarian Situations

The Work of Médecins Sans Frontières

Edited by Jean-Hervé Bradol and Claudine Vidal

The urgency and constraints inherent in certain disasters force Doctors Without Borders/Médecins Sans Frontières (MSF) to take risks or otherwise be resigned to great suffering, disability, and avoidable death. While abandoning ineffective habits and official protocols may lead to the provision of less effective care, cause harm, and squander resources, failing to take the initiative means accepting a critical medical situation.

The authors of this book describe and analyze the emergence of new medical practices in humanitarian situations: in other words, how can we create a momentum for change benefiting affected populations? Taking advantage of lessons learned can help us better understand how to operate in specific settings, with the goal of replacing the non-therapeutic practices that doctors and political decision-makers too often tolerate, citing the poverty and ignorance of affected populations or under the pretext of complying with international recommendations, economic constraints, and public authorities.

This book is a group effort rather than a collection of articles written by experts working independently. The authors are seven doctors, a pharmacist, and three sociologists. They based their work on a review of MSF archives and publications, along with interviews with former and current managers who were or are involved in the process of bringing medical innovation to humanitarian settings.

Chapter 1

Innovation?

Jean-Hervé Bradol and Marc Le Pape

The word "innovation" initially troubled some people at MSF. When we talked to them about innovation, their minds turned to "invention" and thoughts along the lines of inventing a therapeutic drug or diagnostic test. They seemed to doubt that it was possible to attribute such innovations to MSF. Most people think that humanitarian medical intervention is charity medicine using outdated tools—vaccines, diagnostics, and drugs—developed in rich countries that will soon be replaced by a new generation of medical products. Humanitarian medicine is seen as a means of recycling secondhand products for use in precarious situations, not as a source of innovation. Some innovations, though, can even be relevant to resource-rich countries.

Humanitarian medical intervention does often involve simplified treatment protocols, but that does not necessarily mean rudimentary practices. For example, it might mean diagnosing uncomplicated malaria using a rapid test rather than a microscope. Using only a drop of blood on a small test device, rapid tests can confirm or rule out the diagnosis in a few minutes, without a laboratory, and the result can be read with the naked eye by almost anyone. Incorporating the latest advances in immunology, the rapid test is both more sophisticated and simpler to use than the microscope. The innovation in this case has been to implement the new technology systematically across MSF teams. Previously, the lack of a simple test that could be used in precarious situations (large numbers of patients coupled with a shortage of qualified lab personnel) meant treating malaria without laboratory confirmation—in other words, blindly. Unnecessary or inappropriate treatment was therefore administered in proportions that varied depending on the location and epidemiological profile but were sometimes as high as two-thirds of the cases.

Another example of innovation is the fixed-dose combinations that MSF now uses for treating AIDS and malaria. Taking fewer tablets each day improves patient adherence and is part of a successful treatment strategy. Combining several active ingredients into a single tablet, however, is a complex procedure that cannot be improvised: it takes formal research and development to introduce a product with better therapeutic efficacy. These are just two examples of how MSF's medical practice among populations in precarious situations is not "substandard" medicine; in fact, it employs the latest technology and products (medical and surgical) that comply with standards recommended in developed countries.

This suggests that MSF, in keeping with our initial premise, has indeed participated in the process of innovation, and continues to do so—but to prove it we must examine the evidence without illusory hindsight. We recognize the risk, particularly since some of this book's authors have been involved with the organization for many years. Clearly, they cannot observe an organization for which they work as consultants and researchers as if it were any other field of study. Moreover, this examination relies primarily on internal sources, documents, and interviews with MSF participants in the medical programs being analyzed. Drafts of each article were sent for critical review to a group of readers that included other fellow contributors and colleagues from different fields (logisticians, pharmacists, doctors, nurses, sociologists, historians, and political scientists) within the organization.

This approach is in keeping with the self-analysis process by which MSF seeks to identify and build upon important experiences to improve its actions. Since the mid-1980s it has focused, in part, on medical issues (Destexhe, 1987; Brauman, 2000).

Such an approach is expected to improve and advance medical practice by learning from experience. It is also a safeguard against the natural tendency to recall past experiences as a kind of exhilarating, heroic, idealized self-history. Self-examination is not intended to highlight positive actions, but quite the reverse. This is no easy process, and obstacles need to be overcome. Even if risks have been recognized and identified, it is tempting to emphasize the positive results of our interventions. Indeed, glorifying institutional history can distort our perception of humanitarian work, and we must stress here that the improvements in the medical management of the five diseases discussed in this book are the fruit of the collective efforts of many actors and institutions. The contributions of local practitioners, researchers, and health care institutions in affected countries are systematically underestimated. For example, how many people know that it was Niger, the world's poorest country, which developed the international standard for treating epidemic meningitis—not once, but twice, in 1991 and 2005?

Counterexample

In answer to the skepticism about humanitarian medicine's capacity for innovation, we describe a number of treatment protocols (cholera, meningitis, human African trypanosomiasis—also known as sleeping sickness—malaria, and AIDS) the development of which seemed to us noteworthy, positive, and linked to MSF's contribution. These infectious diseases represent a significant part of humanitarian medical activity. New epidemics, increasingly frequent resistance to standard treatments, government perception of infectious diseases as threats to security and economic growth, and commercial and political tensions surrounding access to essential drugs explain, in part, the changes in infectious disease policies in recent years. Though there have been notable advances in other areas of medicine used in humanitarian interventions, they are not dealt with here. For example, psychiatry and clinical psychology have become common practice in the field, and a body of expertise has been developed. To take just two examples from surgery, MSF is now treating fractures by osteosynthesis, or internal fixation, and performing maxillofacial reconstruction. Treatment protocols for women who have been raped have been a major development in gynecology. Pharmacy and laboratory activities have also undergone profound transformation, and we have introduced digital medical imaging in the field. Burkitt's lymphoma was one of the first cancers to have its own treatment protocol for teams in the field.

The five infectious diseases chosen for this book are relative success stories, but this has not always been the case. As a counter-example, we might mention tuberculosis, for which the tests available at our projects fail to establish a diagnosis in half of all cases. The main diagnostic method—looking for bacilli using direct microscopy after staining—dates back to the late nineteenth century. The vaccine, developed in the early twentieth century, is too limited in efficacy to have a real effect on disease transmission, although it does reduce the frequency of some severe forms. The treatment protocol for common forms is too long and too complicated. Moreover, there have been no new antibiotics for treating the common forms since the 1960s, despite the fact that antibiotic-resistant forms—some of them untreatable—have since appeared. The global spread of AIDS—of which tuberculosis is one of the main opportunistic illnesses—has put the prospect of controlling tuberculosis even farther out of reach.

There was an innovative strategy targeting tuberculosis in

the early 1990s. The new approach, called Directly Observed Treatment Short-Course, or DOTS, was based on five main principals: political commitment, microscopy-based diagnosis, continuous drug supply, data collection and analysis, and direct observation of patients taking their medication. The DOTS approach involves a more rational use of existing diagnostic and therapeutic tools, tools that, albeit limited, were at least available. The strategy, which involved humanitarian doctors, was an undeniable advance over earlier practices, but failed to control the disease. It also led to the exclusion of patients not considered important to the overall objective of epidemiological control. This adverse effect underlines the importance of understanding—through careful surveillance prior to embarking on an innovative policy—the new opportunities that a scientific advance is likely to create. It is dangerously idealistic to believe that political will alone, by encouraging caregivers and patients to behave more rationally, can compensate for inadequate science. Not only does the pursuit of unrealistic goals often mean excluding some patients judged non-essential to achieving the (nonetheless impossible) objective—particularly in contexts where there is a paucity of care—but the resources squandered in the pursuit of such illusory goals might have been better distributed.

Case Studies

Malaria

The example of Thailand in the early 1990s (Nosten et al., 2000) involved practical issues (i.e., MSF's participation in malaria treatment trials in several refugee camps). In this type of situation, in order both to recruit cases and follow them, research teams generally work with treatment teams, as shown by the co-authorship of articles in scientific journals. Some of the humanitarian doctors had reservations about participating in the studies. Their objections were based not so much on formal codes of ethics but on general ideological arguments—"patients can't understand," refugees in camps "have no choice," or with relief organizations providing experimental subjects, patients "aren't in a position to give their consent freely." There was also a specific ethical objection to the practice of testing the new protocols successively in the same camps; namely, that the risks of the research were not being distributed equally, but rather borne by a limited number of camps, and concentrated in one population or group. Yet the physician-researchers justified this practice by saying that the refugees derived a direct, immediate benefit from the research, and that access to a new treatment (rather than now-ineffective antimalarials) made them the beneficiaries of what was learned from the studies done on their group—which indeed was true.

Innovation upsets existing relationships between institutions, between practitioners, and between researchers. It produces tensions, shifting alliances, and public opinion campaigns. Each author describes this play of forces and alliances as they reconstruct, in detail, the twists and turns in the innovation process, the arguments from all sides, the actions undertaken, and the political effort expended in forcing the introduction and dissemination of a treatment, a way of organizing care, or a treatment strategy. MSF often plays a specific role in the innovation process, using advocacy to move innovation more quickly from the experimental phase into therapeutic use. Gaining widespread adoption of an innovation also means getting intervention countries to accept a new treatment approach as their national protocol, and working to change public, industrial, and trade policy recommendations. It involves combining medical practice with political action and risking confrontation with the political, economic, and medical powers that be.

With this degree of involvement in the implementation of new treatments, MSF then has to face the consequences. This is where critical self-examination becomes imperative. Once innovations have been proven therapeutically effective, minimalist ethics (Walzer, 1994) and clinical observation consider them a positive thing. But this publicly affirmed belief leads to another, political, one—that innovations can be applied to benefit the whole of society, with positive overall results. So getting new treatments incorporated into national and international health care policies presupposes that the results of applying the protocols on a massive scale will be beneficial. This was MSF's assumption when, in the early 2000s, it recommended that Artemisinin-based Combination Therapy (ACT) be used to treat malaria in sub-Saharan Africa. MSF fought for the acceptance of ACTs into national protocols. But in countries where they are recommended by the Ministry of Health, ACTs have had only a limited effect on the segment with the highest malaria-related mortality (i.e., children under two years). This doesn't mean that introducing ACTs to African public sectors was a bad idea—in many countries they were already being marketed in the private sector. But public health policies being what they are in most African countries, the impact of ACTs remains limited. Those who opposed a wider use of ACTs used this to justify abstaining or simply refusing to introduce them. This absurd argument was used, most notably, by pharmaceutical syndicates[1] in the early 2000s. They claimed that unless all of the conditions necessary for success were in place, simply introducing a new drug would be pointless, and destined to fail.

MSF fought the abstention policy, claiming that for practitioners, correctly treating patients and curing them is never pointless. MSF frequently employs this type of public engagement when introducing an innovation; when confronted with doubts, obstacles, even prohibitions, MSF presents access to new treatments of proven efficacy as intrinsically beneficial

---

1   See Jean-Jacques Bertrand, chairman and CEO of Aventis-Pasteur, and chairman of the *Syndicat national de l'industrie pharmaceutique* (Bertrand, 2000).

and as an objective that cannot legitimately be subordinated to other ends (Dodier, 2003, p. 19–23). Their therapeutic efficacy warrants their immediate introduction. This reasoning bears the unmistakable register of minimalist ethics. It uses arguments regarded as widely, if not universally, understandable, because they generally prompt immediate, spontaneous support: "pretty much anybody looking on will see something here that they recognize" (Walzer, 1994, p. 6). This book presents several examples of how, in the face of powerful opposition, MSF publicly leverages medical ethics to promote its treatment choices and their adoption by international public health institutions and health ministries in intervention countries. This type of debate usually takes place far from the political arena, behind the closed doors of ethics committees. Our investigations show the circumstances under which MSF violates this convention, and the results that ensue.

From a public health perspective, however, the appropriateness of accepting a new treatment and putting it into general use can only be judged by considering overall success. Once judged appropriate, how a new treatment is introduced is dictated by a set of norms formalized and legitimized by the World Health Organization (WHO) and health ministries. Faced with these norms, MSF negotiates, argues, seeks, and finds allies within international institutions, health ministries, and pharmaceutical firms; joins research teams; and, at the same time, engages in overt public criticism of the institutions and companies it believes are blocking therapeutic progress and complicating, or even banning, distribution by public health programs.

Sleeping Sickness

The resurgence of sleeping sickness seems to be under control, at least for now. From the early 1980s to the present, control efforts have been based on the methods and medications of colonial military medicine (with modern medical epidemiological techniques used to refine the targeting of priority intervention zones). Success was not a foregone conclusion. Production of traditional drugs was disappearing, and new avenues of treatment went unexplored. There is no doubt that MSF played an important role in terms of the number of patients treated, attempts to preserve the standard intervention tools (pentamidine, melarsoprol, and mobile teams), efforts to standardize the clinical uses of a new screening test (the card agglutination test for trypanosomiasis), and the development of new treatment drugs (eflornithine and nifurtimox). Beyond the satisfaction of having narrowly avoided catastrophe—an endemic resurgence and no drugs for treating it—a close look at activity in recent years leaves some bitterness. Despite the fact that there has been an alternative (eflornithine) to the standard drug (the arsenic derivative melarsoprol) since the early 1980s, the vast majority of patients treated at Stage 2 of the disease (the neurological stage) were receiving the latter—basically a poison—which not only failed to eliminate the parasite in about one-third of cases, but killed 2% to 10% of patients, or even more in certain series. This means that several thousand patients over the past two decades have died from the adverse effects of the treatment. Practitioners refused to accept this situation, as an alternative existed. We have to remember, however, that these research studies created an ethical dilemma. Conducting clinical trials in which some groups of patients continued to receive arsenic in the early 2000s was questionable. Evidence of arsenic toxicity could have been used to override the methodological imperative of comparing a new treatment (eflornithine and nifurtimox) to the standard treatment (melarsoprol).

In this particular case, standard clinical trial methodology raised questions that the review process and national and international ethics committees do not seem to have considered thoroughly. Then there was the 2001 BiTherapy Trial in Uganda, in which five subjects in the two groups receiving melarsoprol died. What additional information did these five deaths—a predictable response to a treatment that is little more than a poison—contribute to science? Did the aim of comparing a new treatment to an old one that had already failed in a third of cases justify such a high human toll? The clinical trial was modified in the wake of these deaths. In any case, the new treatment has the same implementation problems as the previous one. Unlike specialized teams treating large numbers of cases, bush nurses will have difficulty handling even a simplified injectable treatment safely—as the experience in Ibba, southern Sudan, has already shown. This justifies continuing efforts to research an oral treatment that is effective at both stages of the disease.

AIDS

We should note that there has been a change in political perspective in MSF's arguments. In the late 1980s, the introduction to *Santé, médicaments et développement* (Destexhe, 1987, p. 12) stated: "Research is a long, expensive process that only pharmaceutical companies can afford, and pharmaceutical industrialization of the Third World is not always the panacea." In the early 2000s, however, MSF asserted that research should not be left solely in the hands of pharmaceutical companies, using Brazil's state production of generic antiretrovirals (ARVs) as an example of how to respond to the AIDS pandemic in Africa, where it is taking its most deadly toll. MSF believes that, because of international rules on intellectual property, monopolies held by multinational pharmaceutical companies are among the main obstacles to drug access in low-income countries. And, as noted by Ellen F. M. 't Hoen,[2] the industrialization of what was known twenty years ago as the Third World is now recognized

---

2   http://www.msfaccess.org/main/access-patents/the-global-politics-of-pharmaceutical-monopoly-power-by-ellen-t-hoen/.

as a source of progress in the fight against AIDS: "Most of the ARVs currently available at affordable prices come from India" ('t Hoen, 2009, p. 7).

MSF at first criticized what it considered Third-Worldist utopias, in particular the vision of industrialization projects and the celebration of the "barefoot doctor"—a central figure of Maoist China's health policy which was at the root of public health failures. In the 1990s the organization began to criticize the devastating public health effects of pharmaceutical capitalism. This criticism focused primarily on the considerable advantages—such as patents leading to prolonged trade monopolies—granted to drug manufacturers. MSF commented that as a result, in places where market prospects were poor, entire areas of disease prevention, diagnosis, and treatment were no longer covered by either research for new pharmaceutical products or the distribution of existing ones (Trouiller et al., 2002).

AIDS offered an emblematic example for this criticism at a time when multinational drug companies, governments, and international organizations were in discussions to finalize the intellectual property rules that were adopted in 1994 as the General Agreement on Tariffs and Trade's Trade-related Aspects of Intellectual Property Rights. The dominant trend at the time was to establish a single worldwide price for a drug and drastically limit the possibility of producing it without a patent. Developing nations such as Brazil, India, Thailand, and Kenya, as well as several NGOs, mobilized at the November 2001 World Trade Organization (WTO) meeting in Doha to adopt a declaration asserting the sovereignty of states who were or would be taking public health measures that might include manufacturing and using drugs without the patent holder's agreement (compulsory licensing) and importing drugs already produced at a lower price in another country (parallel importation) without permission from either the intellectual property rights owner or the manufacturer.

What set MSF apart in this context was not that it was making the link between the availability of pharmaceutical products in poor countries and intellectual property issues, but that it was drawing the connection as an international association of doctors publicly testifying that their patients were dying as a result of how the wealthiest countries managed pharmaceutical property rights. MSF's ability to express this opinion simultaneously in multiple forums (gatherings of practitioners and national public health operatives, medical/scientific discussions, WHO and WTO meetings, participation in preparations for the Group of Eight meeting, etc.) was made possible, in the autumn of 1999, by the creation of a specific institutional mechanism—the Campaign for Access to Essential Medicines.

The effect of an approach that couples a demand for flexibility in applying intellectual property regulations with the development of simplified prescribing protocols has been clearly visible: a 99% drop in ARV prices from 1999 to 2007 and an increase in the number of people treated from three hundred thousand in 2002 to three million in 2007 in middle- and low-income countries. However, only a third of patients who need it are now receiving a treatment whose toxicity and limited efficacy have since led to its abandonment by high-income countries. While available data show an increase in the number of people treated, they tell us little about the success or failure of these treatments, which are now prescribed on a massive scale in precarious contexts. Failures are probably more common than suggested by clinical monitoring without laboratory verification (viral load), which is rarely available. Treating more patients or switching drugs to deal with new resistances and reduce toxicity will create new tension around intellectual property issues and increase the strain on program funding.

Meningitis and Cholera

Our critical self-examination should not be limited to studying drug marketing strategies or how we allocate funds internationally for health disasters. We also need to look at the immunization component of MSF's response to epidemic meningitis. MSF has invested massively in outbreak-response vaccination at the start of meningitis epidemics only to realize later that vaccination came too late to have an effect. Research efforts then focused on defining criteria that would allow more timely decisions on outbreak-response vaccination. Yet however sophisticated the data collection, analysis, and transmission tools, the accuracy of the information and the decisions it leads to ultimately depend on the quality of the epidemiological surveillance. Unfortunately, the latter is rarely more efficient than the country's public health structure. So the dilemma is that while the vaccine cannot be used prior to the epidemic due to its short duration of efficacy, it's often not possible to identify a meningitis outbreak quickly enough to use it in time. This would require a public health system that functions well, which is rarely the case. Criticism pointing out the futility of this approach therefore has some merit. Rather than continuing to spend large amounts of money for outbreak-response vaccination yielding meager results, would it not have made more sense to invest in developing a new generation of vaccines that could be used preventively?

A 2007 WHO press release[3] reporting recent developments remained vague as to why progress has been so slow in a field where the science and technology needed for a breakthrough has been available since the early 1990s: "MVP [Meningitis Vaccine Project], a partnership between the World Health Organization (WHO) and the Seattle-based nonprofit, PATH, is collabo-

---

3   http://www.who.int/mediacentre/news/releases/2007/pr28/en/print.html.

15

rating with a vaccine producer, Serum Institute of India Limited (SIIL), to produce the new vaccine against serogroup A Neisseria meningitidis (meningococcus)." MVP director Dr. F. Marc LaForce stressed the project's potential, stating "the vaccine will allow elimination of the meningococcal epidemics that have afflicted the continent for more than one hundred years."

We should add that while meningitis epidemics may be terrifying to the population, they pose little threat to governments, because in the absence of prevention measures governments do not get blamed when people are affected. This makes it easier for the authorities to acknowledge the epidemics, and attention then focuses on the Ministry of Health's response capacity. Not only can the government not be held responsible for the scourge, it can ride to the rescue by organizing mass vaccination campaigns. While epidemiological data do not always support outbreak-response vaccination, the political benefits are obvious. The mass vaccination campaign in 2009 in the northern Nigeria states—usually hostile to what they characterize as intrusion by foreign organizations dangerous to the population's health security—is proof of government interest in immunization against meningitis.

In the case of cholera, MSF's contribution to the standardization of tools, detection, and treatment procedures in closed settings (refugee camps, prisons, etc.) is undeniable. The major challenge in the fight against cholera is in open settings, either urban or rural, where the burgeoning number of small peripheral treatment centers is inevitably accompanied by extra logistics work and greater laxity in treatment supervision—though the latter is crucial to treatment efficacy, particularly in severe cases. The efficacy of the strategy in closed settings rests largely on active detection of cases through health worker home visits, a technique that is easier to implement within the limited confines of a refugee camp. Yet the current cholera pandemic is mainly affecting open settings.

Epicentre[4] studied the feasibility and effectiveness of cholera vaccination and participated in the study of a preventive alternative to reactive treatment alone after the start of an epidemic (Legros, Paquet, Perea, 1999). In 1999 the WHO stated that the oral vaccine (B subunit killed whole-cell, or BS-WC, and rBS-WC) is potentially useful in certain high-risk situations, such as slums and refugee camps (WHO, 1999). Yet despite encouraging results, it will be a long while before those living in areas where cholera is endemic and causes recurrent epidemics will receive vaccine protection. Indeed, cholera, because it highlights the lack of public sanitation services, is no favorite with governments, as demonstrated by the deadly 2008 epidemic in Zimbabwe. Governments often forbid the use of the word "cholera" in both internal public health communications and the press, and there is even greater pressure when the country draws a significant portion of its revenues from tourism.

Despite the fact that it is technically possible to control the disease, there appears little political will to do so. In 2007, for example, the number of cases—underreported for political reasons—was estimated by the WHO at something less than two hundred thousand (WHO, 2008), with some 4,000 deaths reported that same year. By contrast, during the 2007–2008 season, fewer than thirty thousand cases[5] of epidemic meningitis and 2,500 deaths were reported, and two million vaccine doses were administered. Public policy–wise, there is much more effort put toward meningitis—despite the vaccine's limitations—than cholera, even though there are more cholera cases and deaths.

---

4   Epicentre is an MSF satellite organization that specializes in the epidemiology of intervention, research, and training.

5   WHO, *Meningitis Season 2007-2008: Moderate Levels of Meningitis Activity,* July 9, 2008, http://www.who.int/csr/disease/meningococcal/meningitisesepidreport2007_2008/en/index.html.

The disease studies presented in this work show that humanitarian medicine often contributes to medical innovation by first simplifying, then disseminating, scientific and technological advances among neglected populations where such diseases can be catastrophic. The success of this approach rests on influencing public policy. Indeed, when such efforts do not accompany the development of new intervention techniques, medical innovation ends up having little effect on the fate of the poorest. In this domain, the MSF movement—by virtue of its nature and experience—shows greater skill and motivation in the international arena than in national ones, where the association is sometimes viewed as a foreign interloper unacquainted with the subtleties of the local medical and political establishments.

Political and Scientific Vigilance

What does the association see as its responsibility, once the innovations it has championed become accepted medical practice? This is an ongoing source of controversy, even internal crisis. In fact, there is no universally accepted strategy at MSF for dealing with this responsibility. MSF has, however, taken the initiative in ensuring the supply of effective drugs and lowering their cost; for example, MSF-Logistique[6] acts as a drug procurement center for all agencies involved in fighting sleeping sickness.

Clearly, for actions such as these to be in any way relevant, a framework is needed for monitoring and analyzing medical policies on a global scale. There must be specific objectives for MSF involvement when public health is at issue, and MSF must have a clear position before entering public debate.

In particular, political and scientific vigilance allow us to trigger public controversy citing medical work performed during

---

6   On the subject of the MSF satellite organization MSF-Logistique, see the analysis by C. Vidal and J. Pinel in this book.

epidemic crises. The main counter-argument against this advocates examining the consequences of wider use of new health care practices, declares such examination essential to the proper conduct of interventions, and criticizes MSF for not taking this into account, or for doing so in a simplistic, overly hasty manner. MSF usually responds by arguing that treating patients will necessarily have an overall positive effect. Even though its scientific validity remains controversial, this argument—coming from MSF—carries weight in the public sphere when the association engages in critical debates with international institutions (the WHO, United Nations agencies, etc.), donor institutions, drug companies, health ministries, and various institutions from the medical world (scientific journals, specialist groups, etc.). The case studies show that MSF's ability to get the validity of innovations recognized has a lot to do with being there at every stage of the legitimization process: clinical and treatment practices, epidemiology, scientific journals, peer information–exchange (and controversy) networks, analysis, and advocacy. Several chapters of this book describe the framework that permits MSF to intervene in this way in the various areas of legitimization.

While the coherence of this system is essential, its responsiveness also requires individual commitment to remain alert; it is only by this commitment that each person can seize upon new medical tools and treatment strategies that can be imported for use in international emergency responses and transformed by humanitarian practitioners.

However, integrating medical innovation into humanitarian practice also means redefining and rewriting treatment protocols, obtaining administrative authorizations, identifying supply sources, managing the logistical and administrative aspects of pharmaceutical imports, training staff in new practices, closely supervising implementation, and continually evaluating results. In other words, it's a long, demanding process over the course of which initial enthusiasm can turn into exhausting daily uncertainty and, sometimes, disillusionment. When the innovation is a success, its use becomes so routine that hardly anyone remembers how much effort it took to introduce.

Bibliography

Bertrand, J.-J. 2000. "L'industrie pharmaceutique et le tiers-monde." *Le Monde*, May 30.

Brauman, R., editor. 2000. *Utopies sanitaires*. Paris: Le Pommier.

Destexhe, A. 1987. *Santé, médicaments et développement: Les soins primaires à l'épreuve des faits*. Paris: Fondation Liberté Sans Frontières.

Dodier, N. 2003. *Leçons politiques de l'épidémie de sida*. Paris: Éditions de l'Ehess.

Legros, D., C. Paquet, W. Perea, I. Marty, N.K. Mugisha, H. Royer, M. Neira, B. Ivanhoff. 1999. "Mass vaccination with a two doses oral cholera vaccine in a refugee camp." *Bulletin of the World Health Organization* 77 (10): 837–842.

Nosten, F., M. Van Vugt, R. Price, C. Luxemburger, K.L. Thway, A. Brockman, R. McGready, F. Ter Kuile, S. Looareesuwan, N.J. White. 2000. "Effects of artesunate-mefloquine combination on incidence of Plasmodium falciparum malaria and mefloquine resistance in western Thailand: a prospective study." *The Lancet* 356 (9226): 297–302.

't Hoen, E. F. M. 2009. *The Global Politics of Pharmaceutical Monopoly Power. Drug patents, access, innovation and the application of the WTO Doha Declaration on TRIPS and Public Health*. The Netherlands: AMB.

Trouiller, P., P. Olliaro, E. Torreele, J. Orbinski, R. Laing, N. Ford. 2002. "Drug development for neglected diseases: a deficient market and a public-health policy failure." *The Lancet* 359 (9324): 2188–2194.

Walzer, M. 1994. *Thick and Thin: Moral Argument at Home and Abroad.* Notre Dame: Notre Dame Press.

World Health Organization (WHO). 1999. *Potential use of oral cholera vaccines in emergency situations. Report of a WHO meeting (12–13 May 1999).* WHO/CDS/CSR/EDC/99.4. Geneva: World Health Organization.

——. 2008. "Cholera, 2007." *Weekly epidemiological record* 83 (31): 269–284.

Chapter 2

MSF "Satellites"

A Strategy Underlying Different Medical Practices

Claudine Vidal and Jacques Pinel[1]

In the mid-1980s MSF began creating entities that operated independently from headquarters. The first was MSF-Logistique in 1986, followed by Epicentre in 1987, the Campaign for Access to Essential Medicines in 1999, and, lastly, the Drugs for Neglected Diseases initiative (DNDi) in 2003. When MSF-Logistique was created, the organizers wanted to ensure that logistics specialists could prepare for field assignments without being under the direct authority of operational managers. They would then have more freedom for initiative and a more favorable time frame in which to prepare the logistical groundwork for an intervention. MSF has continued this policy ever since.

Has this strategy had repercussions for medical innovation? We offer a brief analysis of the intentions behind creating these satellite entities, and of their effect on working methods in the field.

The intention here is not to reconstruct a history of MSF satellites, determine who initiated these institutions, or describe their development.[2] The objective is to see how MSF built a specific operating culture while expanding its operations. While

---

1   This text is based on interviews conducted with Jean-Hervé Bradol, Rony Brauman, Jean-François Corty, Alain Moren, Jacques Pinel, Bernard Pécoul, Jean Rigal, and Brigitte Vasset.

2   These structures will be called "satellites" throughout the text because, even if they are not all part of the MSF movement, each was the result of an MSF initiative.

the decision to create autonomous entities was in keeping with this culture, and a high value was placed on self-sufficiency, it also stemmed from a changing set of historical factors linked to globalization as well as the historical, geographical, and sociological diversity in the various fields of operation. MSF responded to this diversity by varying its operating methods and accepting a wider range of roles.

Medical care, however, remained paramount, which posed a challenge for MSF: finding the resources it needed to practice medicine in situations and areas with non-existent or poor practice conditions, particularly in refugee camps and wastelands where everything had to be built from scratch. Satellites were created to meet both the ongoing desire for self-sufficiency and the specific requirements of each operation. Lastly, another cultural characteristic is that satellites generally developed their activities based on field experiences and an examination of these experiences by practitioners.

The creation of MSF-Logistique and Epicentre in the late 1980s is therefore based on cultural choices or, if one prefers, on a practical rationale specific to MSF. In return, further developing these satellites helped MSF develop its specific medical practices and often gave the entities the opportunity to be different—and sometimes innovative—when replacing practices deemed ineffective.

It was over a decade after the founding of these first two satellites that the Access Campaign and DNDi were created. These were based on the same principles, but with two differences. Even though they continued to respond to situations in MSF's most common fields of operation, they also tried to act earlier in the process by calling on outside players—mainly those in research and pharmaceutical production—in order to take into account medical shortfalls affecting populations stigmatized as unprofitable. This first difference explains the second: these new entities would, by necessity, initiate and fuel public controversies.

The two generations of satellites differed in focus and approach. For the first generation, in the late 1980s, the key task involved managing internal aspects of operations to ensure quality. Monitoring the technology used in operations or scientifically assessing health conditions required incorporating knowledge, techniques, and skills different from those available at the time MSF was created. This effort was carried out by MSF-Logistique and Epicentre.

In the late 1990s and early 2000s, the second generation of satellites sought to transform the external environment. When it appeared that the vaccines, diagnostic tests, and drugs that comprised the medical kits developed by MSF-Logistique (particularly those designed to fight infections) needed to be replaced, the necessary products were not accessible. This was attributed to a series of obstacles—economic, legal, and political—that would have to be overcome. The association demonstrated the need for these products in their fields of operation and conducted advocacy campaigns based on the ethical obligation to save patients who could be saved if a number of external conditions were changed.

Here, too, other disciplines turned out to be essential to MSF's work. In synergy with the Access Campaign and DNDi, MSF developed relationships with a wide range of organizations, including the World Trade Organization, the Group of Eight, multinational drug companies, patient associations, and health care advocacy groups, with the aim of influencing their policies and initiating new forms of cooperation. Since then, these relationships have played a central role in MSF's political concerns and the controversies in which they have been involved.

The fact that this analysis of the satellites' origins covers a relatively long period should not lead to an illusion in hindsight about any organizational genius specific to MSF. These new structures were based on the dominant practical rationale as well as operational dispositions, as suggested above, and as will be further explored below. If there is anything to be said about MSF's organizers, it is that they did not demonstrate any proclivity for centralization, although they could have. They wanted to avoid excessive expansion of the central apparatus and also expected MSF-Logistique and Epicentre to cover a portion of their own costs through paid services. To highlight this anti-centralist spirit, we will give a brief presentation on MSF-Logistique. Our source, who was instrumental in creating this entity, explains that for three years the organization's leaders simply left him to his own devices. He was then asked to take charge of MSF-Logistique, and this subsidiary relationship has never been called into question.[3]

MSF-Logistique

From Support to Logistics

MSF's expertise has largely been forged by the organization's experience in refugee camps. The first major independent "refugee mission" undertaken by MSF—which, until then, had been working in facilities run by other organizations—was in the Sakeo and Khao I Dang camps for Cambodian refugees in Thailand in 1979. First, the organization developed an intellectual toolkit to understand how the geopolitical context could determine refugees' safety and status. With concerns such

3   The autonomy-of-action principle applied to other newly created institutions. Among them were Liberté sans frontierès (1985); Urgence et développement alimentaire (late 1990s); the creation of MSF sections other than the founding section in the 1980s; and, in 1991, MSF-International, an outcropping of the various sections. It should also be recalled that MSF-Belgium created the Association européene pour le development et la santé (AEDES) in 1984 to expand MSF's involvement in social, public health, and food security efforts; and Transfert, a logistics satellite, now MSF Supply, in 1989. The AEDES cannot be compared to MSF-Logistique because it no longer contributes to the MSF movement.

as these, the operational quality of MSF's missions was initially not a priority. For example, in late 1979, when the number of Cambodian refugees in Thailand rose from thirty thousand to three hundred thousand in just three months, an MSF team was working in a camp (Sakeo) that had only recently opened. Drugs were in boxes piled under a tarp and staff members took whatever medicines were easiest to find. This situation called for the first logistical measure: make drugs available and organize them in such a way that users were able, as much as possible, to understand the various nomenclatures, since the drugs originated from different donor countries. The second measure involved laying the foundations for a procurement system by tasking someone with supplying the medical teams with water and provisions, because the field teams at that time only consisted of doctors and nurses.

In 1980, the Khao I Dang camp housed one hundred thousand refugees. There were also other camps along the Thai–Cambodian border. The MSF team, numbering forty to forty-five members, was staying in a small town that they left every day to work in Khao I Dang and other camps. A logistical system was needed, even if it was only rudimentary. In addition to the physical organization of the pharmacy, lists of drug orders corresponding to the various diseases were created and sent to the doctors, who were required to follow procedures. It was also necessary to set up a car system, to know who needed to go where, and to make sure that staff put the keys on the board for the next person. There was obviously nothing novel about these measures in themselves, but they were completely new to MSF medical staff.

Every day, a doctor and two nurses would go to one of the border camps, where five thousand to then thousand refugees were taking shelter. Each camp included a clinic where women could give birth and a drug storage facility. MSF could, if necessary, receive authorization from the Thai military to evacuate patients to the Khao I Dang hospital. Some of these camps served as rear bases for combatants wanting to liberate Cambodia from Vietnamese occupation, however. The Vietnamese would attack and destroy the camps, people would flee into the forest, and everything would be looted. The camps might then become inaccessible for several days. So MSF had to call the military every morning to find out whether the medical team could enter the camp where it was scheduled to work. When the answer was affirmative, the team could only remain for two hours. This meant deciding what to take and then preparing it, a process which led to time-wasting debates.

There was no systematic solution to this problem. Nevertheless, even though the team could not know in advance what it was going to find on site, the camps' medical situation was not unknown. There were women ready to give birth who might need to be evacuated. Other patients had injuries, respiratory infections, and malaria that needed attention. A standard toolkit appropriate for this general situation was created: a large box made by local carpenters that could serve as an examination table and that contained emergency kits and drawers in which supplies were classified by need. Time was no longer wasted when team members left for work because all they had to do was to put the box in the back of the truck. The box was called "semi-mobile equipment" because it was heavy and cumbersome. Several boxes were made, and each one was assigned a manager to ensure that it was kept up-to-date. Several copies of a document with the protocols of five or six diseases were included; this document was developed by the International Committee of the Red Cross (ICRC), which coordinated the medical teams working in the Khao I Dang camp.

The MSF teams in Thailand grew to include 110 people working at nine camps. They added experience at the national level to the skills they had already acquired in the Sakeo and Khao I Dang camps. A standard nomenclature was now used to order drugs, a manager was responsible for the cars, and an administrator was assigned to each team.

This system, introduced in 1980, seems rudimentary in hindsight, and indeed it was. Yet the fact remains that it heralded a decisive change in the way MSF perceived its organization. It now associated the effectiveness of its medical humanitarian work in emergency situations with logistics specifically designed for such situations—logistics that could be deployed quickly in response to supply and transport needs, along with communications between teams and headquarters. It took several years gradually to identify and resolve the major difficulties stemming from the integration of medical activities and logistical skills. In 1986, the decision was taken to give the teams working on these issues autonomy to set up a satellite—and thus was born MSF-Logistique.[4]

A special study would be necessary to provide a detailed analysis of how the association between medicine and logistics produced specific organizational methods, and how these methods evolved as MSF's activities rapidly expanded during the 1990s. A number of the practices and technologies adopted relied on existing models, but they were streamlined based on field experience and integrated in such a way as to remain consistent with the entire system.

MSF's innovation was to become independent in practical matters by creating its own protocols and tools. It was necessary to set up multidisciplinary teams of medical and non-medical staff. Logistical specialists quickly became essential to these teams,

---

4   MSF-Logistique was formally established in Mérignac in 1992. At the beginning, it was explicitly modeled after the Central Procurement Unit at the United Nations Children's Fund (UNICEF). In addition to drug procurement, field operational logistics and technical support (energy, cold chain, vehicles, etc.) were also developed, which made MSF's medical operations more efficient.

even giving rise to "another" medical position (Diaz, 2006). Moreover, to maintain a balance between old and new medical players, MSF had to accept the fact that the usual medical hierarchies would not necessarily be reproduced in the field. Because medical personnel with practical experience in these regions were essential for the success of these missions, young physicians could exercise responsibilities that would normally be performed by department heads in their own countries, and nurses could take over medical management of a mission.

Kits and Guides

The semi-mobile equipment was the first in a series of kits designed by MSF. It was not itself an invention, having been modeled on techniques used by the French emergency medical service. It was, however, an embryonic innovation because it was part of the specific "ecology" of emergency humanitarian interventions: a large number of patients from poor communities facing precarious security conditions and typically living in unfavorable and hard-to-reach areas, combined with a high turnover of medical personnel, most of whom had no experience with the tropical diseases they now had to learn how to treat.

In Thailand, the Office of the United Nations High Commissioner for Refugees (UNHCR) drafted an emergency medical guide in the early 1980s. Oxfam designed a nutritional kit. MSF teams revised the guide based on their own experience to anticipate responses to situations in which it would be used. This became the Clinical Guidelines. Standardized drug and equipment lists were drawn up and everything, including user manuals, was packed into kits intended to meet the needs of ten thousand people for three months. The Clinical Guidelines was called the "green guide," after the color of its cover. Together with the kit, it was expanded and revised by its users when they reviewed any of its chapters.

A guide to essential drugs was added to the green guide. It was designed for medical staff with very different levels of training: for doctors unfamiliar with tropical environments, for nurses, and for national doctors working with MSF. At the outset, the guides and kits met the need for streamlining operations management, but they also sought to standardize medical practices. Combined with MSF's training program and operating culture, the kits turned out to be effective and applicable to many emergency situations. In 1988, the World Health Organization (WHO) put a label on the kit, calling it the "new emergency health kit." Some advocated retaining the MSF label. Others pointed out that the WHO's endorsement made it more influential, even if it had largely been developed by MSF. Since then, the International Committee of the Red Cross (ICRC) has become a major purchaser of the green guide for its operations. Furthermore, the kit has often been "borrowed"—which is to say, illegally translated—in various countries with MSF's tacit approval. Its first editions, in fact, arrived in the field with "Please copy" printed on the endpaper.[5]

Since the "historic" kit created in Thailand, MSF-Logistique has created many other kits. To cite one example, the vaccination kit for measles, meningitis, and yellow fever enables MSF quickly to set up a cold chain and includes all medical and logistics supplies necessary for a vaccination campaign by several teams of vaccinators. The surgical kit, which contained resources allowing medical personnel to perform three hundred operations and manage one hundred hospital patients, includes drugs, renewable supplies, and the necessary equipment to meet the needs of an existing hospital's surgical program. There is also a kit for creating a hospital with inflatable tents.

---

5   "The first WHO guides, whose content was rather scientific, were not operational guides. And, if you read the WHO guides now in MSF's areas of expertise, nearly all of them are copy-and-paste versions of MSF guides. In my opinion, what seems to have changed international practices is the fact that MSF guides are created in the field; not a single one comes from a review of the literature." Interview with Alain Moren (epidemiologist and currently project manager at Épiconcept, Paris), November 2006.

While this type of kit was unquestionably inspired by military medicine, there are major differences between military surgery and the type of surgery practiced by humanitarian organizations. Military surgery as practiced by wealthy countries is much more sophisticated but gives priority to treating a more limited population—wounded soldiers. Even though the two concepts are close, in practice the MSF kit's composition is different. It has enabled advance planning for surgery in humanitarian situations and has provided rapid intervention capacities under satisfactory technical conditions that previously existed only within the militaries and civil defense services of developed countries' militaries.

Lastly, a three-fold imperative—consistency, simplification, and learning from experience—drove the process carried out jointly by MSF and its logistics satellite. In order for a kit to meet the needs of a given humanitarian situation, the supplies must be consistent with the operating method recommended in the reference documents, training must conform to these documents, and at least one or two team members must have experience in comparable situations. In the early 1980s, MSF practitioners were concerned about the continual loss of field expertise due to high staff turnover. This concern provided powerful motivation for producing the first guides.[6] While even those guides may have seemed presumptuous given MSF's modest experience, they were the best way to preserve and enhance field experience.

Epicentre

The effort to improve medical practices in response to emergency situations relied on the ability to codify and

---

6   "When I went to Cameroon, I brought lots of books with me and an encyclopaedia of surgical techniques, which had cost me 10,000 francs. They rotted from the humidity, but I had thought I would need them. The lack of possible referral was frightening. We had nothing. So I was happy to write, simplify, and transfer [knowledge]." Interview with Jean Rigal (currently Medical Department director, MSF-France).

develop standards and to provide the elements necessary for conducting field operations. Through this normative process of preparing supplies appropriate to the circumstances, the teams could develop micro–working environments in contexts where it would not otherwise have been possible to conduct medical activities effectively.

In addition, any emergency operation inevitably involves risk-taking, even if a highly detailed understanding of the situation helps limit risk. This risk culture, adopted and controlled to the extent possible, was transferred to the medical arena. MSF doctors made recommendations that they felt were better suited to their patients' living conditions and that they had the logistical means to implement. But these recommendations sometimes met with resistance from national or international medical authorities. At other times, recommendations that could be carried out in one region were rejected in another. Lastly, and most frequently, these recommendations concerned a large number of patients. As a result, it was considered essential to set up a system of epidemiological assessments and surveys in tandem with the development of a logistics system.

MSF officials then decided to create subsidiaries based on several disciplines—medicine, biology, statistics, and more—in order to conduct research and epidemiological activities. The aim was to provide scientific support to operations and sell epidemiological assessment services to other organizations. At the time, developing training and methods for the type of assessment sought by a practitioners' association was an innovation in itself (a medical computer expert was even added to the Epicentre team in 1987). As with logistics, MSF decided to allow these specific professions, which differed from MSF's core activities, to operate according to the principles of their own fields of expertise. And thus, Epicentre was created.[7]

Epicentre's strength is the ability to apply epidemiology quickly in crisis situations. This rapid response, which did not exist outside MSF,[8] was made possible by MSF-Logistique. It was still necessary to come to a decision and create the opportunity. In fact, it was rare for a team to manage the requirements of a daily research project that did not come into play during the operation itself and did not appear to be a priority. Experience gradually won over the players in the field when, for example, epidemiological data validated the introduction of a single-dose injectable or oral drug to replace a one-week treatment.[9]

The Campaign for Access to Essential Medicines

Epicentre's creation reflected an aspect of the operating culture that was developed during the 1980s: trying to find upstream solutions to improve patient treatment, taking into account the specific needs of practitioners in the field. The Access Campaign, created in 1999 and based on the same rationale, was also set up as a subsidiary of MSF. There was more to it than that, however: the Access Campaign took on, albeit for its own specific objectives, a role regularly assumed by MSF—that of a "witness" engaged in political advocacy. The Access Campaign therefore worked from the beginning with human rights and health care activists.

In 1996, MSF and Epicentre organized an international colloquium for the purpose of exposing and condemning the lack of medicines necessary for treating infectious diseases—a worsening situation that was striking developing countries

---

7   See Emmanuel Baron's study in this book.

8   It should be recalled that in the United States, the Centers for Disease Control and Prevention's concept of intervention epidemiology had explicitly served as an example.

9   "MSF Epicentre is almost unique because, other than MSF, there is no other NGO capable of doing research in the emergency situations in which it operates." Interview with Alain Moren.

particularly hard.[10] The speakers noted that while rich countries had achieved significant progress in all medical fields, humanitarian organizations were increasingly unable to respond effectively to epidemics for the following reasons: the production of certain drugs had been abandoned because they were not considered profitable by pharmaceutical firms (in the case, for example, of human African trypanosomiasis—also known as sleeping sickness); other drugs were no longer effective due to resistance developed by parasites (the chloroquine-resistant malaria parasite, among others) and no research was underway to discover new treatments; overly restrictive treatment protocols that were difficult to comply with and encouraged the appearance of resistance that left the patient without any recourse; and antibiotics that were effective but unaffordable.

Different levels of responsibility were identified: systems for protecting brand-name drugs that prevented the production of much cheaper generic drugs; the utopias endorsed by international organizations (the WHO and UNICEF) such as the program "Health for All in 2000," which relieved states of their duty to provide medical care; pharmaceutical companies' lack of interest in researching and producing medicines for disadvantaged populations; and the priority given, even by MSF, to prevention rather than treatment.[11]

Some MSF management no longer accepted that they had no choice but to provide increasingly poor treatment or no treatment at all, and wanted the quality of care in crisis situations to become one of MSF's priorities. First, a Medicine Unit was created within MSF-France in 1997, followed by a Research Group on Essential Medicines.

---

10   "Operational responses to epidemics in developing countries," Lariboisière Medical School, October 25, 1996.

11   "Out of 1,233 innovative drugs sold from 1975–1997, only 11 targeted a tropical disease" (Trouiller, 2000).

The Medicine Unit, initially consisting of only a few people, understood that other types of expertise had to exist alongside pharmacological and medical skills, especially legal knowledge of the patent system. The treatment of certain diseases also needed to be simplified in order to broaden and improve implementation, particularly by MSF. The unit realized that it had to appeal to public opinion worldwide by conducting systematic campaigns, but these campaigns required solid information based on the work of consultants and experts across a wide range of fields. Various disciplines were eventually grouped together in a separate body called the Access Campaign, which became a subsidiary as an MSF inter-sectional project, thereby giving it broad scope.

The Access Campaign achieved results by leveraging MSF's reputation—the organization was awarded the Nobel Peace Prize in 1999—and its "ability to make itself heard." The following recollection by one of the Medicine Unit's members serves as an example. He recalled that a letter protesting the abandonment of an essential medicine (eflornithine) for the treatment of sleeping sickness had not received any response from the manufacturer. A few years later, the company resumed production and MSF received free supplies of the drug on condition that it manage the global stock and handle distribution.

MSF thus developed a strategy of operational independence in terms of logistics, scientific assessment, and advocacy for the production of essential medicines. This development resulted in a decision to avoid depending on other organizations. The emergence of different medical practices resulted indirectly from this policy of autonomy. This policy also prompted a gradual transformation in the role played by MSF physicians, who increasingly became both practitioners and promoters of new medical procedures, as evidenced, for example, by MSF's conflicts with the WHO. MSF called for changes in protocols and new therapeutic strategies and criticized treatments and products it deemed ineffective, even when the WHO and national medical authorities continued to endorse them.

DNDi

A press release issued in Geneva on July 3, 2003, announced that five prestigious medical and research institutions were joining forces with MSF to create DNDi.[12]

Developing drugs from existing compounds was one of the main ideas motivating the partners to create DNDi. When the major pharmaceutical companies lost interest in tropical diseases, they had already developed compounds for potential medicines but had not yet reached the final stages. It was therefore necessary to conduct clinical studies, but that is not one of MSF's activities. Several universities had conducted, and continued to conduct, basic research on neglected diseases and had discovered molecules without developing them into drugs. The companies could have used this research, but they lacked interest because it involved reportedly unprofitable markets. DNDi took the position that the development of new treatments for the most neglected diseases could not result from market incentives and that a public commitment to meeting these needs was required. It was therefore necessary to mobilize a network of institutions in agreement on this type of research and development strategy.

Medical innovation plays a key role in DNDi, and it could have a considerable effect on treating diseases that affect

---

12   "The six organizations are the Indian Council of Medical Research, Pasteur Institute (France), the Kenya Medical Research Institute, Médecins Sans Frontières, the Ministry of Health of Malaysia and the Oswaldo Cruz Foundation (Brazil). WHO/TDR will participate in the meetings of the Scientific Advisory Committee of DNDi as an observer to provide expert scientific and technical advice as required. DNDi will work in close collaboration with the UNDP/World Bank/WHO Special Programme for Research and Training in Tropical Diseases (WHO/TDR) to achieve its goals." DNDi press release, "Best science for the most neglected: Creation of a new not-for-profit drug research organization," July 3, 2003, Geneva.

massive numbers of people in the southern hemisphere. For example, in the case of sleeping sickness, which is one of DNDi's priorities, the development of an oral tablet to treat the two forms of the disease without being too toxic would be a radical change for patients.[13]

Some at MSF consider DNDi a fundamental and innovative break with the past: neglected diseases can now be treated. One member, speculating how MSF might be perceived in a few decades, thought that people may one day forget its pioneering role as a medical organization, but not DNDi or its "invention" of a new political economy of drugs. Is this a utopian view bound for disillusionment? Perhaps, but without a touch of utopian idealism, how can we practice the "impossible discipline of innovation" in medicine (Latour, 2003)?

For more than two decades, the creations of structures that are autonomous yet retain an organic link to MSF's medical activities have contributed to improving the quality of its operations. The studies in this book of certain diseases provide detailed examples. But contributions from satellites also weaken MSF's crippling tendency to rigidly and endlessly reproduce its operating culture. By inviting contributions from those who have acquired experience outside MSF and have had professional relationships with a wide range of institutions, MSF's satellites bring in a range of perspectives on humanitarian medicine. Their contribution is not limited to developing logistical or medical tools, producing scientific assessments, or trying to remove obstacles to necessary, but inaccessible, drugs. As intermediaries, they draw MSF into dialogue in many different settings, encouraging the association to open up and learn from others.

---

13   See Jean-François Corty's study in this book.

Bibliography

Diaz, F. 2006. "Les 'autres' métiers de la santé. Le logisticien humanitaire." *Sèves* 10: 43–50.

Latour, B. 2003. "L'impossible métier de l'innovation technique." In *Encyclopédie de l'innovation*, P. Mustar, H. Penan, 9–26. Paris: Économica.

Trouiller P. 2000. "Médicaments indigents." In *Utopies sanitaires*, R. Brauman, editor, 195–205. Paris: Le Pommier.

Chapter 3

Measure, Analyze, Publish, and Innovate

Emmanuel Baron

MSF stepped up the pace of its activities in the early 1980s. More interventions meant recruiting more staff and developing more technical and logistical resources. The perceived image of a responsive, efficient medical relief organization intervening in violent situations all around the world was confirmed. The general public had little doubt about the grounds for MSF's decisions to intervene in particular situations and the effectiveness of its actions. After all, it was argued, MSF's contribution was better than nothing: providing care, by definition, does no harm. Media coverage increased accordingly, with intense exposure when the organization took a public stand on a particular situation—for example its expulsion from Ethiopia in 1985.[1]

This dynamism in the field was coupled at headquarters with an urge to see the organization acknowledged as a credible entity in the medical and scientific community. While MSF was highly regarded by many, the organization's practices smacked of medical exoticism. Little of any tangible value in medical and scientific terms seemed likely to come from this pleasant team of doctors: while their good intentions were not in doubt, some saw them as cowboys, others as boy scouts, and this, along with their limited technical resources, inevitably placed them on the

---

1   In October 1985 MSF-France denounced migration forced by the Ethiopian authorities. The majority of other relief organizations did not take a public stand and made no plans for a withdrawal. MSF received an expulsion order two months later.

margins of scientific rigor and medical progress.

There was a need for the organization to be more rigorous and more efficient. For some, this meant developing internal resources that would allow the organization to generate more independent analysis, scientific output, and training methods. What MSF wanted at the time was to be able to describe and measure its activities without relying on staff and input from other institutions. Its decision to learn, master, and develop quantitative measurement methods applicable to the programs it ran and the situations in which it operated was in some sense a way for MSF to shed the lingering impression that it was a collection of newcomers rather than a serious medical organization.

To this end, MSF looked to skills being developed and taught primarily in the United States. American universities had, in fact, long since developed research and training programs in epidemiology, the public health discipline that describes, quantifies, and analyzes the situation of particular populations and patients. Several MSF doctors went to the US to be trained in epidemiology and played a part in planning a structured project that was being drawn up at the organization's headquarters.

Epicentre was created as a French non-profit organization in 1987. Its status was that of an independent organization, although its board of directors was made up primarily of members of MSF. Its name is based on the broad notion of a center of energy and the term "epidemiology," the discipline that underpins its actions. Its initial aim was the same as it is today: namely, investigating critical situations in the field, in particular population displacements and epidemics; carrying out research on behalf of MSF in the areas in which it operates; and training medical personnel in epidemiological techniques.

Epicentre's position in relation to MSF—as an internal organization and yet a distinct entity—is in itself unusual. It is more common for international research institutes to be independent from operational organizations. It was because of its original organic relationship with MSF and its medical practice, freed from the ever-uncertain task of seeking external funding, that Epicentre was able to anchor itself in the realities of the situation in the field and build its capacity for scientific output.

This position would help it to formulate, in scientific terms, the practical constraints facing medical teams. The human and geographical environment in which MSF operated complicated such basic medical questions as, for example, diagnosing malaria without risk of error. Epicentre was able to assess difficulties of this kind and translate them into describing constraints on interventions, then into research, and sometimes even into international health issues. Taking a population census, comparing strategies and treatments, and measuring their effects all rely on a knowledge base that is constantly changing but has largely been developed in relation to stable, defined environments. Because MSF was engaged in humanitarian interventions in countries with inadequate health care facilities and with populations that were often on the move and of an uncertain size, Epicentre was placed in a scientifically challenging situation.

Stimulated by the pace of relief operations, Epicentre was able to support MSF in its choices at three levels: defining its intervention priorities; changing its practices; and sharing its experiences.

Measuring and Analyzing to Define Priorities

Epicentre's main role initially was to describe, measure, quantify, and compare different situations. MSF's programs were most often set up without the benefit of any health-risk indicators. Experienced volunteers had an intuitive understanding, based on their work in the field, which enabled them to mobilize resources and take action using their collective familiarity with general field conditions rather than an analysis of the quantitative data specific to a given situation. Making objective measurements of the characteristics of different health situations—the difficulties of providing relief, and their successes and failures—helped to highlight the constraints under which MSF teams were operating. It was this scientific analysis of tangible situations that drove the move towards innovative research.

This sequence (data collection–analysis–need–innovation) proved relevant in meningitis epidemics, the operational response to which consists of treating the sick while vaccinating those not yet ill. The large number of people requiring treatment (several thousand) and vaccination (tens or hundreds of thousands, and even several million in Nigeria in 2009), and the fact that the population is scattered are significant constraints. Traditionally, describing an epidemic relies on gaining access to information about timing (how long has the epidemic been going on, how many cases are there by unit of time?); location (where are cases occurring in geographical terms?); and people (what kind of patients are affected, particularly in terms of age?). Quantitative descriptions of these events by teams in the field and graphic representations of them are both ways of assessing the number and geographical origin of cases, the time taken for MSF teams to intervene, the proportion of patients who have died in hospital, and the resources mobilized. Epicentre has investigated several such epidemics in Niger, Burkina Faso, Sudan, and Nigeria. An analysis of the information gathered combined with the teams' assessment of their own work, and particularly of the difficulty of providing antibiotic injections over several days, helped to highlight the need to cover a broader proportion of the population affected and to have access to a simpler, shorter treatment regime to cure a larger number of cases. Based on these observations, MSF and Epicentre carried out comparative clinical trials in West Africa, the results of which confirmed the effectiveness of therapy based on a different injectable treatment administered in a single dose. In using well-known, tried-and-tested methods to quantify MSF's action in the field in the areas where it operated, Epicentre was not doing anything particularly innovative. But it was able to translate the constraints and consequences of mass treatment and vaccination into scientific language, thus helping a consensus to emerge in favor of alternative solutions.

Epicentre also used quantitative methods in the context of armed conflicts. During the 1980s, MSF frequently worked with displaced or refugee populations fleeing violence and assembled in more or less organized camps where they waited for help from non-governmental organizations or United Nations (UN) organizations. The precariousness of their physical and psychological state, and the conditions in which they had settled and were living, required a rapid deployment of medical and non-medical assistance. This was split into roughly ten priorities for action, which were supposed to reduce the risk of major levels of morbidity occurring within the population. Similar priorities had already been outlined in the late 1970s by the Centers for Disease Control and Prevention in Atlanta in relation to conflict situations, but they needed further consolidation (CDC, 1992). Using population survey methods that had been tested elsewhere—although never on a large scale in this type of context—Epicentre was able to shed light on general health indicators such as the incidence of certain pathologies, immunization levels, and mortality rates. These data were an indication of the vulnerability of the populations that MSF was assisting and provided the necessary basis for establishing the actions that should take priority in relation to health (Brown et al., 2008).

MSF's work with the Kurds in Iraq is a good example of Epicentre's contribution to relief activities. In 1991 MSF deployed human and medical resources on a significant scale to

43

support a population fleeing in chaos and panic from the threat of the Iraqi army, then finding itself on the Turkish border, unable to escape. In one of the largest operations in the history of MSF, epidemiologists from Epicentre were dispatched and quickly gathered information that enabled them to describe the health situation and send relief to where it was needed most.

Epicentre thus confirmed the effectiveness of using methods that offered a swift estimate of health indicators for a given population on a large scale. Using these methods in the international context of responding to catastrophic situations—which would become a routine practice—provided essential quantitative data for establishing the gravity of such situations and an objective basis for organizing assistance. In fact, Epicentre's work has become a benchmark in the world of humanitarian assistance (even if some surveys lacked rigor, were limited in methodological terms because they were carried out too late, or were not always adequately exploited by the operational staff who requested them.) In a document published in 2007 by the Humanitarian Practice Network[2] and designed to summarize existing information and recommendations for key players in the field of international humanitarian assistance, eighteen of the sixty-two bibliographical references were for research carried out by Epicentre and MSF.

Field studies routinely include questions on the conditions in which they have been carried out and on subsequent use of the results obtained. The complex environment in which these surveys are conducted needs to be taken into account to assess the validity and reliability of the measurement techniques used. Describing a health situation on the basis of calculating a rate that shows a risk means knowing the number of people exposed to that risk or the rate at which particular events, such as death,

---

2   The Humanitarian Practice Network is a forum run by a British organizsation, the Overseas Development Institute, a think-tank on humanitarian action and development policies

occur. The accuracy of such estimates is questionable when populations are unstable and migrating because of threats and violence. The very structure of these populations varies when, for example, young men become the victims of atrocities and disappear. The indicators produced are therefore subject to these kinds of uncertainty. Methods do exist to limit the effects, but the point is still the subject of discussions in several publications (Working Group for Mortality Estimation in Emergencies, 2007; Checchi, Roberts, 2005). Although the necessity and use of such surveys has not been called into question as such, the debate has gone so far as to cause public controversy, in particular around the publication by American researchers at Johns Hopkins University in Baltimore of an estimate of the number of deaths attributable to the invasion of Iraq by the US Army (Roberts, 2004; Burnham, 2006).

This issue was highlighted in late 2009 when the Health Nutrition Tracking Service—an inter-agency partnership set up under the aegis of the World Health Organization (WHO)— asked Epicentre to produce a critical review of mortality and nutritional surveys carried out between 2006 and 2008 in North Kivu, an area in the east of the Democratic Republic of Congo that had been the scene of intense fighting for some fifteen years (Grais et al., 2009a,b). From roughly thirty reports that tackled the question of mortality and nutrition in the region, four were selected on the basis of a list of criteria examining the methods used, results obtained, and their subsequent use. Each used different methodologies. Three had been carried out for the purpose of effectively targeting relief, while the fourth was designed to communicate to the public what the population was suffering. This research also highlighted the fact that, even if this kind of survey was based on tried-and-tested methods, questions could be raised around how they were applied. Furthermore, they are sometimes carried out too late to have any real influence on how relief is deployed.

There has also been lively discussion about operational teams' motivation for requesting field studies. More precisely, the issue at stake was the use of the results: was their purpose to target actions more effectively, or to make a public statement about the situation the population was living in, which humanitarians felt was intolerable?

In the first case, the dilemma comes from the weight operational managers give to the figures when they compare them with a subjective assessment of the situation. In Chad in 2007, for example, there was a discussion within MSF on the significance of the high mortality rates obtained in a survey carried out among displaced Chadian and Sudanese families in the Ouaddaï region, close to the border with Sudan, and to the Darfur region in particular. The people who had requested the survey were MSF operational managers, who compared it with their first-hand assessment of the situation when setting up the relief program. The criticism that arose at MSF was that too much faith was being placed in the survey for fear that action would only be taken on the basis of the statistics. Although in this case the criticism did not completely reflect the reality of the facts and the decisions taken, the argument is still valid for other situations.

In the second case, the initial motivation for a survey may be public advocacy. Figures may be used in unintended ways by those outside the organization, however. The most emblematic example is that of Somalia in 1992, when the results of an Epicentre mortality survey on the displaced population were used, based on a false interpretation of the results by senior officials within the UN, to help justify the *Restore Hope* operation—led by the US Army—with its well-known consequences.

Measuring and Comparing to Change Practices

Over the years, through Epicentre, MSF became increasingly accustomed to using quantitative methods for health assessments in emergency situations. The knowledge it gained opened up other ways of assessing its actions. Populations in precarious situations and morbid phenomena such as epidemics were therefore not its only areas of research. Epicentre was also involved in research activities designed to improve medical treatment per se, and to measure, compare, and evaluate new diagnostic and therapeutic strategies in relation to standard practices.

MSF medical managers dealing with a number of conditions postulated that some of the diagnostic or therapeutic techniques being used were not the most effective or easiest options, or that others could be applied in situations where they were not yet in use. The treatment of meningitis was a good example, but work was also done on other pathologies that caused MSF problems, even real dilemmas: examples in the 2000s included malaria, human African trypanosomiasis (sleeping sickness), tuberculosis, and malnutrition.

Malaria: The Relationship Between Research and Political Decision-Making

In the late 1990s, chloroquine was still the standard treatment for malaria in Africa. Even then, there were clinical and parasitological indications that strains showing resistance to the treatment and responsible for fatal forms of the illness were becoming increasingly prevalent. Inspired by experts in the field and academics who had already described the same phenomenon in Asia, MSF decided to commit to widespread use of a combination therapy based on artemisinin derivatives in its program. The treatment, known as Artemisinin-based Combination Therapy (ACT), was well known and used in Asia

(China, Vietnam, and Thailand, primarily) and was based on the principle of the synergy between two anti-malarial drugs (one of which was an artemisinin derivative) which acted in complementary ways. The treatment struggled to gain a foothold in Africa because of the medical and political authorities' mistrust of new products, which were more expensive than the previous generation, and because of the relatively poor data available to confirm that chloroquine was no longer effective. MSF asked Epicentre to carry out a number of studies designed to confirm that chloroquine was not effective enough to be prescribed without endangering patients suffering from malaria. Support within MSF for carrying out studies of this kind was not unanimous. Some of the organization's former senior figures argued that this was an overly technical and ultimately pointless approach to a situation to which the response was self-evident. The argument certainly made sense: it was reasonable to suggest that chloroquine was already less effective than previously thought and also to assert that the refusal of the national authorities in one particular country had more to do with other interests than public health concerns or the absence of concrete scientific evidence. Conversely, others argued that empirical decisions in a medical environment should make way for processes that lead to a rigorous demonstration of the efficacy of therapeutic choices. A consensus finally emerged for launching a series of surveys based on MSF programs. The results unambiguously supported a switch to combined therapies and were echoed in the thrust of MSF's Campaign for Access to Essential Medicines under the slogan "ACT Now." The results were also published in internationally recognized scientific journals (Guthmann et al., 2008). By verifying the comparative efficacy of two therapeutic strategies in children suffering from malaria, Epicentre provided part of the argument for the political battle being waged by MSF.

Despite the publication of basically conclusive results, the issue did not end there. Some countries took time to agree to the change in their national protocols. Furthermore, not all sections of MSF moved at the same pace in changing medical protocols. This resulted in some tense discussions, particularly in the case of Burundi, where some sections accepted the government's delay in implementing the new recommendations, thereby placing their medical personnel in one of the most uncomfortable positions a doctor can face: namely, prescribing a treatment with a very high likelihood of failure.[3]

Sleeping Sickness: The Relationship Between Research and Standards

Results from Epicentre's clinical trials on sleeping sickness have contributed to significant progress over previous treatment recommendations. For fifty years, patients at the advanced stage of the illness had been treated with a drug (melarsoprol) derived from arsenic, the efficacy of which was decreasing due to the emergence of resistant strains of the parasite responsible for the disease. In addition, the treatment was so well known to cause death by damaging the brain that some infected patients refused to undergo screening for the illness. The only other drugs available were not officially recommended and of doubtful efficacy as a single treatment (nifurtimox), or difficult to administer (eflornithine). Furthermore, large-scale use of eflornithine on its own as a front-line treatment raised the threat of the parasite developing resistance. Conscious of the limitations of the existing treatments, but above all because there were no other therapeutic options available, MSF and Epicentre decided to carry out a clinical trial to compare the efficacy and tolerance of the three drugs in a combined therapy (melarsoprol–nifurtimox, melarsoprol–eflornithine, and nifurtimox–eflornithine). The supposed advantage of these combinations was that they

---

3   See the studies by M. Le Pape and I. Defourny, and S. Balkan and J.-F. Corty in this book.

could enhance the way in which each drug acted and avoid natural selection of the resistant strains of the parasite.

The initiative was opposed by a number of specialists in the illness, including at the WHO. Their accusations centered on the failure to comply with drug development rules. Good practice and standards in this area would, indeed, have meant going through some lengthy stages, and would have necessitated testing the three combinations of drugs in different doses, *in vitro* and *in vivo*, and not carrying out trials on patients until a later stage of the development process. MSF and Epicentre would be seen as behaving like sorcerers' apprentices if they did not follow the requirements of each stage.

Epicentre and MSF managers put forward other arguments to justify their intentions. In addition to factors associated with the declining efficacy of melarsoprol and the absence of any other back-up solution in the medium term, the standard development process would delay the availability of a potentially effective solution for several years, while the situation demanded an immediate response. Their intention was to test several options and conduct the trial on the basis of a rigorous methodology, including the involvement of an independent monitoring committee which could stop the study should it be deemed ineffective or one of the combinations prove toxic. While they did not obey standard procedures to the letter, MSF and Epicentre thought they were complying with them in spirit. They were supported by several national program managers in the countries concerned.

The trial started in Uganda, in partnership with the Ministry of Health, in 2001 in consultation with French and Ugandan ethics committees. The monitoring committee swiftly decided to interrupt the trial after 54 of a planned 435 patients had joined, because of the higher than expected number of deaths in patients on a combination of melarsoprol and nifurtimox. The deaths did not call into question the basic principle of combination therapies, but were a harsh reminder of what was already known about the limitations of melarsoprol. The study was published; the combination of nifurtimox and eflornithine seemed promising in light of these albeit only partial results (Priotto et al., 2006). A process had been set in train and led MSF and Epicentre to do further research into this combination, still in Uganda, on a second series of cases (Checchi et al., 2007). Following further encouraging results, hopes of abandoning melarsoprol increased. Epicentre then embarked on a large-scale, multi-center trial designed to compare the efficacy and innocuousness of a combination of nifurtimox and eflornithine in a shorter (from fourteen down to ten days) and simpler treatment (number of drips cut by three-quarters) than with eflornithine alone, another standard treatment. This was met with the same reticence from the scientific community: MSF and Epicentre were failing to comply with traditional drug development procedures and were running the risk that nobody would support the use of this combination even if effective and well-tolerated. It was better, so the thinking went, to take the time required for the usual processes to guarantee future recognition and acceptance of possible positive results by the health care professionals and authorities concerned. Preferring to maintain the momentum they had built up, and confident of the results they had already achieved, MSF and Epicentre embarked on a larger trial that was also supported and co-financed by the Drugs for Neglected Diseases Initiative (DNDi).[4] This trial, conducted from 2003 to 2008 at four separate sites in the Congo Republic and the Democratic Republic of Congo, confirmed what had been expected: the new combination was shown to be just as effective and well-

4   DNDi was founded in 2003 by a number of private and public sector partners (including MSF, the Institut Pasteur, Indian Medical Research Council, etc.), in order to fill the gaps in terms of research, development, and recording of neglected tropical diseases (see the study by C. Vidal and J. Pinel in this book).

tolerated as treatment with eflornithine alone at a high dose. The results were presented at scientific conferences such as the American Society of Tropical Medicine and Hygiene in New Orleans in December 2008 and published in 2009 (Priotto et al., 2009). The inclusion of this combination in the WHO list of essential drugs in 2009 marked an important step in the hoped-for amendments to the national protocols of the African countries concerned. There is still a long way to go, however, between demonstrating the superiority of a treatment and large-scale production, followed by registering it with the authorities, and finally its routine use in dispensaries and hospitals.

Tuberculosis: The Relationship Between Research and Scientific Inertia

Meanwhile, AIDS continued to kill through so-called opportunistic diseases, which gain a foothold because of the patient's weakened immune system. One of these is tuberculosis. MSF had long been involved in treatment programs for the disease. One of the obstacles facing medical teams, however, was ensuring proper diagnosis. This relied on old methods and the limited effectiveness of microscopic isolation of the bacillus responsible for the illness in the sputum of patients suspected of having damage to their lungs—the most common clinical form. According to international recommendations, tuberculosis treatment, which lasts at least six months, means isolating the bacillus at least twice in three successive sputum samples over two days. If the results are negative, which is common among children and patients infected with the HIV virus, treatment can be instigated on the basis of a set of clinical and radiological criteria. These procedures mean patients have to travel to treatment centers and involve a significant workload for the laboratory. Following an internal discussion, supported by experts from the University of Liverpool and the Kenyan Medical Research Institute, and based on data from a study carried out in 2005 in Nairobi to assess a microscopic diagnostic technique using concentrated sputum samples, Epicentre was able to evaluate a simplified strategy for diagnosing pulmonary tuberculosis based on one rather than two positive sputum samples. This simple reduction was just as effective, but made it possible to diagnose two-thirds of patients with the disease at their first consultation, reduce the number of laboratory tests by a third, and avoid losing touch with patients while waiting for their test results (Bonnet et al., 2007). In 2007 these results contributed to the change in the WHO's recommendations for microscopic diagnosis of tuberculosis.

Although this type of research is evidence of a refusal to accept the status quo, MSF and Epicentre nonetheless again found themselves obliged to carry out research designed to improve unsatisfactory diagnostic techniques for tuberculosis although their effectiveness did not, in fact, change radically. This is because MSF is at the end of the chain, and thus only "picks up" old techniques; even a minimal change to these seemed to represent an advance. Indeed, there were few new avenues in tuberculosis diagnosis or treatment suggesting any significant changes likely to improve patient care in the near future. There seemed to be few options for practitioners and patients in the countries of the South, where there is little scope for using sophisticated molecular biology techniques. Alongside its research and scientific papers, MSF added a public communications campaign, which it hoped would raise awareness among key players and funding bodies involved in public policy. In 2003, MSF's Campaign for Access to Essential Medicines published a document setting out the resources and prospects for tuberculosis diagnosis and treatment (Access Campaign, 2004). The illness had been completely neglected in terms of research and solutions, and future prospects did not look at all promising. The epidemic had spread, and the situation for patients had been getting worse for decades in the face of a somewhat indifferent attitude on the part of public authorities, manufacturers, and medical officials. The public campaign that accompanied the report gave MSF the opportunity to denounce this situation by explaining the serious difficulties it was facing in treating more than twenty thousand new cases each year. While new research is now being pursued within a context of public–private research and development partnerships, and while the WHO's message on treatment strategies for patients is less dogmatic than it was, there is still a shortage of momentum. MSF's position has changed little since then, while the focus of Epicentre's research and its commitment remain the same.

Malnutrition: The Relationship Between Research and Programs

Although it works in the field alongside MSF, Epicentre has not always agreed with the pace of operational priorities. In some situations, the relationship between MSF and Epicentre has been strained. This was the case when treating malnourished children in Niger in the early 2000s. MSF, the Campaign for Access to Essential Medicines team, and Epicentre disagreed at the time on the principles of their respective missions. The conflict was between those who lobbied to prioritize assessing the demand for operational innovation, those who believed in the need to communicate the emergency in necessarily simplistic language, and those who wanted to take the time needed to carry out an effective analysis of the effects of operational choices. Members of MSF who were advocating a change to nutritional protocols wanted data and analyses that would support their point of view. This was where they ran into a lack of understanding from Epicentre, which was focused on managing the constraints around scientific output in unstable areas and the issues that should be subjected to scientific analysis in relation to emergency relief. This example of internal tension within MSF, between groups whose roles and objectives should ideally work in synergy, resulted in the publication of a number of scientific articles (Isanaka et al., 2009).

Publishing Scientific Data

Since its creation, Epicentre has been expected to publish its research. Public dissemination of the methods used and results obtained is an integral part of scientific research. It is based on a codified process, the result of which consists of presenting, in a concise and well-argued manner, the essential details of the investigative methods used and the results gathered and analyzed, followed by a discussion of their validity. Epicentre was thus expected to engage in the exercise of scientific writing. Initially, several pieces of research were communicated in the form of letters to the editor of the British scientific journal *The Lancet*. Since then, the number of articles has increased: no fewer than 250 were published between 1988 and 2008, mostly in English.

An example of Epicentre's ability to translate MSF's operational decisions and their effect on the treatment of patients into scientific language was published in *The Lancet* in April 2006 (Ferradini et al., 2006). This study tried to assess the efficacy of antiretroviral (ARV) combination therapies on a sample of a cohort of HIV-positive patients accepted into a treatment program run by MSF and the Malawian Ministry of Health in the rural district of Chirazulu. This was an innovative project, primarily because of the high prevalence of the disease, the rural environment, and the use of a combination therapy in a single pill, a formulation that did not exist as such in developed countries at the time. The results showed that, in patients who had received more than six months of treatment, the presence of the virus in the blood, measured by its viral load, had fallen to a very low level. This figure suggested, among other things, that this form of treatment had an effect on patient survival. These results confirmed MSF's operational choices and Epicentre, which had taken responsibility for conducting the study, could ensure they were published in a scientific journal.

A key principle of the submission process prior to publication is a critical peer review of the manuscript. But appropriating and generalizing from the results of Epicentre's research by any other player in the private or public sectors would have been pointless unless they were rigorously expressed, even if in a very standardized way. It could certainly be argued that the cost of access to scientific journals tends not to favor scientific advances being made universally available, but in fact, the reasons for the lack of recent progress in the diagnosis and treatment of tropical diseases lie elsewhere. There have, however, been some moves towards other editorial models, based on free access to published articles.

Moreover, the editorial process highlights the primacy of channels that are certainly accessible, but which do not always reflect the realities of scientific progress. It is possible to see the effect of a final validation method, a sort of obligatory final stage, although the subject is known and has been discussed and covered extensively in forums, conferences, and journals with a more limited distribution. Sleeping sickness is a good case in point. In 2008, Epicentre reported on five years of work on the treatment of sleeping sickness by giving short presentations at a number of international conferences.[5] A similar observation can be made on new treatments for malaria or the results of ARV treatment programs for HIV-positive patients in the countries of the Global South. Oral communications, or more informal forms of dissemination at meetings of experts, including within the WHO, are often a preliminary to the formal publication process. Epicentre has always made use of these unwritten rules.

Since its creation, Epicentre has sought to establish relationships in both the public and private sectors. It has always seemed

5   In South Korea, at the International Congress for Tropical Medicine and Malaria; in the Democratic Republic of Congo; to the scientific and political authorities of the countries affected by the disease; and in the United States, at the conference of the American Society of Tropical Medicine and Health.

quite normal to monitor changes in medical and scientific knowledge and thus identify the main avenues being pursued by other international medical research teams. It is difficult to assess the direct effect of this function, but Epicentre's decisions to embark on new areas of research has at times clearly had as much to do with its observations on where the gaps lay in the international agenda as the operational constraints being faced by MSF.

Through Epicentre, epidemiology has played a significant role in providing relief in the areas in which MSF operates. The nature of Epicentre's relationship with innovation is twofold: its integration into the MSF organization makes its work easier, but it is caught up in the rhythm of operations and their constraints.

Initially, introducing the techniques of descriptive epidemiology into work in the field was an innovative move. New light was shed on operational issues—where and how to act—and medical constraints—how to diagnose and treat. The transfer was not simply about reproducing a technology in exactly the same way, however; constant work was needed to adjust and refine quantitative measurement methods. The use of these methods and the results produced have been an ongoing source of criticism and debate.

The next step was MSF's decision to propose the adoption of new medical practices. Epicentre embarked on studies on which MSF relied in the area of humanitarian medicine, which can be classified as a "latent area of science" (Kourilsky, 2006). Acquiring the techniques and language of science enabled MSF to propose the adoption of new medical practices and to be heard on occasion by both its peers and the public health authorities.

Epicentre's use of epidemiology cannot be dissociated from the choices made by MSF in terms of medical policy. In fact, Epicentre has to reconcile the rigor of a scientific process with the specific constraints of humanitarian situations and the requirements expressed by the organization during the course of its actions. It is within MSF, as an integral part of its activities, that Epicentre has to confront the dilemmas inherent in the relationship between caring practices and scientific activities in sometimes extreme situations. There is no easy way of resolving these dilemmas: the judgment made depends on the political choices involved in the decision.

Bibliography

Bonnet, M., A. Ramsay, L. Gagnidze, W. Githui, P. J. Guerin, F. Varaine. 2007. "Reducing the number of sputum samples examined and thresholds for positivity: an opportunity to optimize smear microscopy." *The International Journal of Tuberculosis and Lung Disease* 11 (9): 953–958.

Brown, V., P. J. Guerin, D. Legros, C. Paquet, B. Pécoul, A. Moren. 2008. "Research in Complex Humanitarian Emergencies: The Médecins Sans Frontières/Epicentre Experience." *PLoS Medicine* 5 (4), e89.

Burnham, G., R. Lafta, L. Roberts. 2006. "Mortality after the 2003 invasion of Iraq: a cross-sectional cluster sample survey." *The Lancet* 368 (9545): 1421–1428.

Campaign for Access to Essential Medicines (Access Campaign), Médecins Sans Frontières (MSF). 2004. *Running out of breath? TB care in the 21st century.* Internal report.

Centers for Disease Control and Prevention (CDC). 1992. "Famine-affected, refugee, and displaced populations: Recommendations for public health issues." *MMWR Recommendations and Reports* 41: 1–76.

Checchi, F., L. Roberts. 2005. *Interpreting and using mortality data in humanitarian emergencies. A primer for non-epidemiologists.* Network

Paper 52. London: Humanitarian Practice Network.

Checchi, F., P. Piola, H. Ayikoru, F. Thomas, D. Legros, G. Priotto. 2007. "Nifurtimox plus Eflornithine for Late-Stage Sleeping Sickness in Uganda: A Case Series." *PLoS Neglected Tropical Diseases*, 1 (2), e64.

Ferradini, L., A. Jeannin, L. Pinoges, J. Izopet, D. Odhiambo, L. Mankhambo, G. Karungi, E. Szumilin, S. Balandine, G. Fedida, P. Carrieri, B. Spire, N. Ford, J.-M. Tassie, P. J. Guerin, C. Brasher. 2006. "Scaling up of highly active antiretroviral therapy in a rural district of Malawi: an effectiveness assessment." *The Lancet* 367 (9519): 1335–1342.

Grais, R. F., F. Luquero, E. Greletty, H. Pham, B. Coghlan, P. Salignon. 2009a. *Forest for the Trees: A critical review of rapid surveys conducted in North Kivu, 2006–2008*. Report to an expert committee at the World Health Organization.

Grais, R. F., F. Luquero, E. Greletty, H. Pham, B. Coghlan, P. Salignon. 2009b. "Learning lessons from field surveys in humanitarian contexts: a case study of field surveys conducted in North Kivu, DRC 2006–2008." *Conflict and Health* 3 (1): 8–13.

Guthmann, J.-P., F. Checchi, I. Van den Broek, S. Balkan, M. Van Herp, E. Comte, O. Bernal, J-M Kindermans, S. Venis, D. Legros, P.J. Guerin. 2008. "Assessing Antimalarial Efficacy in a Time of Change to Artemisinin-based Combination Therapies: The Role of Médecins Sans Frontières." *PLoS Medicine* 5 (8): e169.

Isanaka, S., N. Nombela, A. Djibo, M. Poupard, D. Van Beckhoven, V. Gaboulaud, P. J. Guerin, R. F. Grais. 2009. "Effect of Preventive Supplementation With Ready-to-Use Therapeutic Food on the Nutritional Status, Mortality, and Morbidity of Children Aged 6 to 60 Months in Niger: A Cluster Randomized Trial." *Journal of the American Medical Association* 301 (3): 277–285.

Kourilsky, P. 2006. *Optimiser l'action de la France pour l'amélioration de la santé mondiale. Le cas de la surveillance et de la recherche sur les maladies infectieuses.* Report to the French government. Paris.

Priotto, G., C. Fogg, M. Balasegaram, O. Erphas, A. Louga, F. Checchi, S. Ghabri, P. Piola. 2006. "Three drug combinations for late-stage Trypanosoma brucei gambiense sleeping sickness: a randomized clinical trial in Uganda." *PLoS Clinical Trials* 1 (8), e39.

Priotto, G., S. Kasparian, W. Mutombo, D. Ngouama, S. Ghorashian, U. Arnold, S. Ghabri, E. Baudin, V. Buard, S. Kazadi-Kyanza, M. Ilunga, W. Mutangala, G. Pohlig, C. Schmid, U. Karunakara, E. Torreele, V. Kande. 2009. "Multicentre randomised non-inferiority trial of nifurtimox-eflornithine combination therapy for second-stage gambiense sleeping sickness." *The Lancet* 374 (9638): 56–64.

Roberts, L., R. Lafta, R. Garfield, J. Khudhairi, G. Burnham. 2004. "Mortality before and after the 2003 invasion of Iraq: cluster sample survey." *The Lancet* 364 (9448): 1857–1864.

Working Group for Mortality Estimation in Emergencies. 2007. "Wanted: studies on mortality estimation methods for humanitarian emergencies, suggestions for future research." *Emerging Themes in Epidemiology* 4, 9.

Chapter 4

Controversy as a Policy

Marc Le Pape and Isabelle Defourny

MSF is no stranger to controversy. Indeed, the organization does not view controversy as negative, but rather as an engine for change. Here we present two recent examples of innovative medical practice where MSF was involved in controversies and used them to its advantage. The controversy originated within the MSF movement; the organization then found itself in disagreement with national authorities in the countries where it operated, international institutions such as the World Health Organization (WHO), the World Bank, the United Nations Children's Fund (UNICEF), pharmaceutical companies, governmental agencies and/or donor organizations—particularly the United States Agency for International Development (USAID)—and renowned specialists in medicine, epidemiology, and the economy. The two examples we have chosen concern the treatment of malaria in Burundi and of malnutrition in Niger.

Conflicting opinions created powerful constraints on validating improved treatment protocols and therapeutic strategies. Different and rival validation processes were suggested. We will describe the different stages of the controversy and the people involved (Lemieux, 2007). Likewise, we will illustrate the connections between experimental demonstration, humanitarian medical practice, and the different forms of public and political involvement.

Malaria in Burundi: The Introduction of Artemisinin-Based Treatments[1]

The Beginning of the Controversy (2000–2001): Therapeutic Requirements

On December 12, 2000, MSF published a press release in Paris, Brussels, and Geneva entitled "Malaria epidemic in Burundi: MSF teams are dealing with an unprecedented influx of patients. MSF demands support from the WHO for more effective treatments." This warning was based on data from sixteen health centers at which MSF was working, as well as on a retrospective mortality survey conducted between October 13 and December 9, 2000, which found "worrying levels of mortality." The press release described MSF's curative and preventive initiatives "from the beginning of the epidemic," and indicated factors "favoring" the sudden increase in the number of cases and the high mortality rate. Three factors were identified: the development of swamp farming; the abandonment of anti-vector policies; and the "probable high resistance to chloroquine." The press release ended with an appeal to the WHO and the Roll Back Malaria (RBM) network—a WHO initiative created in 1998 associating UNICEF, the United Nations Development Programme (UNDP), the World Bank, and other private and public partners to fight malaria (Packard, 2007, p. 217–227)—to "support the use of artemisinin-based treatments."

The press release was the first public expression of dissent. There was no divergence of opinion regarding the incidence of malaria, however: to underline the "dramatic" increase in the number of cases, the WHO, in its recommendations, had

---

1   See the chapter written by S. Balkan and J.-F. Corty. It describes the development and initial use of these treatments in Southeast Asia. We use the term Artemisinin-based Combination Therapy (ACT) to designate therapeutic drug associations based on artemisinin derivatives.

referred to an MSF survey of three health centers (Kassankogno, Allan, Delacollette, 2000).[2]

The controversy began in November 2000, but was not made public at the time. The desk officer responsible for programs in Burundi stated at the MSF board meeting of November 17: "Sadly it is currently impossible for us to use artemisinin derivatives because the government has asked us 'not to introduce any new drugs.' All efforts to secure support from the WHO have proven fruitless because the organization will not recommend the use of medicines that are not registered in the country. This is a sad example of the ongoing struggle to use the best available treatments."

MSF sparked controversy amongst its peers on the following issues:

- Criticism of policy. In general, the WHO should not base its advice on local government policy as this hinders diagnostic and therapeutic progress.
- The choice of treatment. At the beginning of November 2000, MSF recommended the use of artemisinin derivatives combined with sulfadoxine-pyrimethamine (Fansidar) for the treatment of uncomplicated malaria in Burundi. For complicated malaria cases, MSF recommended artemether (Paluther) combined with sulfadoxine-pyrimethamine. These choices were justified by the therapeutic efficacy of the treatments, a lower rate of transmission, and the reduction in the development of resistance. Furthermore, artemether was on the WHO's list of essential drugs, which should have facilitated its introduction.

---

2   The malaria epidemic was unusual for several reasons. It occurred in the Burundian high plateaus, a zone where malaria is not usually present, and a very large number of people were affected. Epicentre performed retrospective mortality studies in three provinces that estimated 1.5 million cases and sixteen thousand deaths in these provinces alone for the epidemic of 2000–2001 (Guthmann et al., 2007). Figures of thirty thousand deaths and 3 million cases appear realistic for the seven affected provinces. Burundi has a population of 7.5 million.

- The fear of high resistance to sulfadoxine-pyrimethamine developing if used as monotherapy in response to the epidemic. On November 16, the WHO began to recommend the use of sulfadoxine-pyrimethamine (replacing chloroquine) as first-line treatment for uncomplicated cases.
- The need to conduct chloroquine and sulfadoxine-pyrimethamine resistance studies in Burundi, as prescribed by WHO protocols.

The RBM coordinator initially replied to these fears, criticisms, and proposals by email over the RBM network on December 13, then again the following day in a public document in which the WHO justified its recommendation for the treatment of uncomplicated malaria (i.e., replacing chloroquine with sulfadoxine-pyrimethamine). Sulfadoxine-pyrimethamine was to be prescribed as monotherapy, without combinations with other anti-malarials.[3] Three justifications were made:

- Therapeutic efficacy. Studies conducted in Rwanda and Tanzania were cited as proof.
- Operational constraints. Burundian medical staff were already familiar with this treatment, and it was available in large quantities in Burundi and elsewhere in the region.
- Observance of treatment, facilitated by the extremely simple single-dose regimen.

The authors of the WHO report explained why they did not recommend a combination of sulfadoxine-pyrimethamine and artesunate as first-line treatment, despite recognizing its efficacy. They referred to the lack of available data in Africa, the problem of adherence to treatment, and the fact that artesunate

---

3   WHO, *Burundi—Malaria epidemic, Treatment choices*, December 14, 2000.

had not been registered by Burundian health authorities. But one development was announced in the document: the Ministry of Health had adopted artemether for the treatment of severe malaria. Earlier, in an internal document, the WHO had already recommended artemether as second-line treatment, but only "if it is registered in the country" (Kassankogno, Allan, Delacollette, 2000).

In his communication of December 13, the RBM coordinator added that even if the therapeutic efficacy could justify the use of an artesunate–sulfadoxine-pyrimethamine combination, a series of factors specific to the situation in Burundi led to problems with its use, including: difficult access to patients, the lack of qualified medical staff, and the absence of stocks of the drug in the region. The MSF desk officer conducting the discussions in Paris was quick to address the issues over the network Website, focusing on the effectiveness of sulfadoxine-pyrimethamine. According to resistance surveys conducted in two Rwandan health centers in 1999 and 2000 by the WHO, the drug was effective in only 64% of cases at the first site and just 53% at the second site. The officer added that this data, as yet unpublished, had been communicated to MSF by the WHO. He was therefore less optimistic than the WHO about sulfadoxine-pyrimethamine monotherapy. Its use on a massive scale would accelerate the development of resistance. He reaffirmed the arguments in favor of artemisinin-based treatments, arguments already presented to the RBM network and publicly stated by MSF on December 12.

The MSF author went on to stress several points in his response:

- Burundian patients were already used to taking treatment over several days—conventional chloroquine treatment lasts three days—so there was no reason to believe that observance would be more problematic with the MSF-recommended regimen.

65

- Artesunate had already been introduced into Burundi. It was available in pharmacies in Bujumbura, and was also registered as a medication reimbursed by the civil servants' health insurance. Treatment protocols, however, were often inadequate. Its inclusion in the national malaria protocol, at least during the epidemic period, would reduce the risks of uncontrolled prescription.

- The logistical and professional constraints were real, but MSF field experience in three provinces showed that the epidemic zones could be reached using mobile clinics. As to the lack of specialized staff, the MSF author took a practitioner's stance: why would the medical staff, already familiar with three-day chloroquine–sulfadoxine-pyrimethamine treatments, not be able to adapt to the three-day artesunate–sulfadoxine-pyrimethamine treatment?

- Supply of the new drug was a significant problem, but MSF declared it was prepared to supply artemisinin derivatives if they were accepted by the Ministry of Health. The objective was to introduce artemisinin-based combinations "at low cost." It should be noted here that the MSF author broached the economic side of the problem, but without explaining how to obtain low-cost combinations, or comparing the costs of the different treatments proposed.

- Medical necessity (the term ethics was not used): although it was perhaps not possible to introduce artesunate everywhere in Burundi, it should at least be introduced where possible. Not all patients would be accessible, but some at least would receive the correct treatment.

The "treatment choices" document published by the WHO on December 14, 2000, did not put an end to the controversy. At the MSF France board meeting on December 22, the Burundi epidemic was back on the agenda. The medical and logistics experts involved at headquarters noted that the debate ("essentially via email and the WHO RBM debating site") "had the effect of modifying WHO recommendations that now include the treatments we advocate (using artesunate), but stop short of recommending them for first-line treatment."

MSF therefore continued to criticize the first-line treatment recommendations, notably in a letter published in *The Lancet* in March 2001 (Gastellu-Etchegorry, Matthys, Galinski, White, Nosten, 2001). This letter was signed by two MSF medical directors and three medical researchers specialized in malaria. The authors described using combinations including artemisinin derivatives as an "ethical obligation," as they were the most effective treatments available. They added that this ethical obligation applied not only to doctors, but also to NGOs and international agencies. The authors therefore asked that the WHO and donor agencies recommend the "immediate" use of these treatments.

In April 2001 the WHO adopted a new protocol recommending the use of combination therapies, preferably ACTs, for first- and second-line treatments in countries with proven resistance to standard monotherapies (WHO, 2001). These were general recommendations, and it was up to individual states to integrate them into their national protocols. The decision was taken in Burundi in July 2002, and implemented some months later in 2003.

Conflict with the Burundian Ministry of Health (2001–2002): An Ethical Obligation

The French section of MSF began using ACTs in 2001, even though the Burundian Ministry of Health did not recommend them for the treatment of uncomplicated malaria. Local health authorities were informed, and tolerated this practice until October 2001, when MSF-France decided publicly to denounce the treatment protocol for uncomplicated malaria, unfavorably comparing the poor results of the national protocol with artemisinin-based treatment data obtained from one of their programs in Kayanza Province. The Health Ministry replied by demanding the withdrawal of ACTs from all health centers where MSF was active, then, shortly afterwards, on November 8, decided to suspend all MSF activities in Kayanza Province for two months. In mid-December, the Burundian authorities expelled MSF-France's head of mission from the country.

The general director of MSF-France wrote to Burundi's health authorities and the WHO to justify localized introduction of the new treatment. The letter, dated November 9, was also sent to high-ranking members of the RBM network. It listed all the organization's arguments, emphasizing the therapeutic efficacy of the new treatment. Medical officials in Burundi nevertheless continued to implement a protocol (sulfadoxine-pyrimethamine monotherapy) that MSF practitioners in the field had noticed was no longer working. MSF believed the national protocol could no longer be respected, and decided to start using an artemisinin-based combination "immediately" without waiting for the results of assessments by the Ministry of Health and the WHO. This is also why "volunteers were sent to the field with supplies of artesunate and amodiaquine." The letter brought ethical obligations to the forefront, stressing that a doctor is obliged to administer effective treatment, and affirming that MSF respected this obligation in Burundi, as it did elsewhere in the world. Our analysis here does not seek to determine whether this level of rigor was, in 2001, universally practicable and practiced by MSF, but we note that theory and practice were coherent in Kayanza Province. For Burundi, this was a challenge to national sovereignty. It is thus understandable that the controversy escalated into a crisis, as each camp claimed to act on fundamental principles, which only served to intensify the disagreement. In the end, only a meeting between the

Burundian president and the presidents of the MSF international movement and MSF-France resolved the crisis. At the end of the talks, the Burundian president asked MSF to continue working in Burundi.

In March 2002, several MSF senior staff members met with the WHO director general, who agreed to support the transition to artemisinin derivative–based treatments, but reminded them that the WHO was a decentralized organization, and that the African branch did not agree with the policy. She stressed that the United States also expressed strong opposition to the use of ACTs .

The escalation from disagreement to crisis had repercussions within the MSF movement. From November 2001, MSF-France asked the three other sections working in Burundi, "Why are we the only MSF section in this mess? How are you treating uncomplicated malaria?" The controversy within the movement intensified and spread on January 16, 2002, when a letter entitled "Are we alone?" was sent—in French and English— by the Parisian desk officer for Burundi "to all MSF sections, their presidents, general directors, operations directors, desk officers and program managers." The letter not only suggested an appropriate strategy for Burundi, but also for generalizing the new treatment and bringing the whole MSF movement into the process. The issue was to address "the question of malaria treatment in general in Africa" and to start a public campaign to obtain approval and use of effective treatments for "all populations" in countries affected by chloroquine and sulfadoxine-pyrimethamine resistance. According to the author, this position should be publicly adopted by all MSF sections, adding: "Who is prepared to stand up, speak out and act?"

The letter sparked strong emotions within the MSF movement, and created a confrontation essentially on the following question: what is the best strategy to trigger change in the national protocol in Burundi? The author sent the letter to all senior MSF decision-makers; this tactic was denounced as bypassing the usual decision-making procedures in order to get the French section's strategy approved. Some opponents stressed that the Parisian position was in line with general agreement throughout the movement on the necessity to change such protocols. They explained that the French section was in no way fighting the battle on its own, but that it had isolated itself in Burundi through the strategy of confrontation it alone had adopted; it was simply being brought back to order and to reality. Others denounced MSF-France's self-glorification: the section gave the impression that they alone were fighting for the right protocol. The criticisms were based on the belief that there was a more effective strategy than confrontation: a strategy involving "silent diplomacy," working to convince, and intervening at all levels with all involved parties. This alternative approach was seen as the best way to help change the protocol.

When the Burundian government agreed to a change of protocol, the process of dealing with disagreements between the different sections finally returned to its normal course, through institutional regulation.

Economic Constraints

MSF's first public interventions only rarely mentioned the cost of ACTs. Nothing was mentioned in the press release dated December 12, 2000, and only a passing reference was made in the article published in *The Lancet* in March 2001: "We appreciate the considerable operational and economic obstacles involved in changing national malaria policies, but there is an ethical obligation ..." (Gastellu-Etchegorry, Matthys, Galinski, White, Nosten, 2001).

But MSF did not neglect the problem of the cost of ACTs. Initially, the issue was not a matter of public debate, but it was discussed within the organization and in exchanges with the

WHO and the Burundian authorities. MSF-France's medical and logistical director declared at a board meeting in December 2000 that "we hope to bring the price down to one dollar," without explaining how he might go about it. In an October 2001 letter to Burundian parliamentarians, the general director of MSF-France admitted that cost "is a major difficulty" and added that MSF was committed to "finding solutions," comparing the situation with that of the treatment of AIDS patients. At the beginning of 2002, once the necessity to change to ACTs in general in Africa had been recognized—particularly for countries with high levels of resistance to sulfadoxine-pyrimethamine and chloroquine (Guthmann et al., 2008)—MSF began to focus on overcoming the financial obstacles. This became evident during the annual meeting of the East African Network for Anti-malaria Treatment. On February 13, 2002, in Nairobi, MSF published a report entitled "Changing national malaria treatment protocols in Africa. What is the cost and who will pay?" The report presented a cost assessment for changing the protocols in five African countries (including Burundi). Its author declared that the change would be too costly to be borne by the governments involved and would require international funding. This sparked another lengthy controversy involving NGOs, donor agencies (particularly USAID), and international institutions. The focus was on the search for solutions to guarantee both a drop in the cost of ACTs, and their supply.

In September 2008, the director of the Global Fund to Fight AIDS, Tuberculosis and Malaria declared that an economic mechanism had been established that should, from 2009 onwards, allow the sale of ACTs in pharmacies at an equivalent cost to chloroquine in countries with endemic malaria. The mechanism requires the Global Fund to invest $150 million to $300 million yearly.[4]

4   "Michel Kazatchkine: "When the world gets together, we get results," *La Croix*, September 9, 2008.

Severe Acute Malnutrition:[5] From Treatment to Prevention

Between April and June 2005, MSF published three press releases in Paris on the gravity of the "nutritional crisis in Niger" and described its response to the problem. None of the three press releases mentioned the word "famine."

On April 26, 2005, MSF reported an "abnormally high" number of children suffering from severe acute malnutrition admitted to their inpatient and outpatient facilities in Niger. The association called for urgent "general food distributions," without indicating who should be responsible (other "aid actors" were mentioned, but without giving details).

A second press release, on June 9, 2005, highlighted the fact that twice as many children under five had been admitted to MSF nutritional programs as in 2004. The report was based on a nutritional survey performed by MSF and Epicentre at the end of April 2005. Unlike the preceding press release in April, the June 9 press release clearly stated a demand for a new general policy and that "exceptional measures must be undertaken urgently." MSF called for food distributions so that "the most vulnerable populations can gain direct, free access to food." MSF also introduced provocative elements in its public communication, criticizing the inadequacy of Nigerien government operations ("sales of moderately priced cereals"). It called for the "mobilization of donors and of international organizations such as the [United Nations World Food Programme (WFP)] and UNICEF," as the only way to provide free food distributions. The call for help was accusatory: stating that these institutions needed to mobilize was to say that, until then, they had been failing their mandates.

A third press release was published on June 28. The urgent need to act was reiterated, but more forcefully: "there will be

---

5   For criteria defining severe acute malnutrition see WHO, UNICEF, *WHO child growth standards and the identification of severe acute malnutrition in infants and children,* Geneva, 2009.

thousands of avoidable deaths this summer." MSF continued to denounce "the reluctance of donor agencies and the government to provide free food distributions," as they "obstruct appropriate relief efforts." However, the press release also had a singularly practical approach compared with previous ones. MSF's president took a practitioner's stance when he stated, "easy-to-use nutritional products adapted for children now exist, that save lives in a few weeks of treatment." Neither of the two previous press releases mentioned this therapeutic argument, clear even to those that know nothing about the treatment of malnutrition and the debates on free food distributions.

Many controversies have arisen on the treatment of infanto-juvenile malnutrition in Niger and some are still ongoing (Olivier de Sardan, 2008). In 2005, the controversy intensified, transcending the medical domain to become a political crisis. We will not give an account of all the twists and turns, nor the diversity of positions taken. The collective work edited by Xavier Crombé and Jean-Hervé Jézéquel (2009) provides a description of the different levels of controversies and public commitments that characterized the crisis. The most visible debates could be qualified as political, economic, sociological, epidemiological, and medical.

Here we describe two controversial aspects of MSF's action: first, free food distribution; and second, the introduction of new nutritional products associated with the change in therapeutic strategies.

The Therapeutic Innovation Predates 2005

At the end of July 2001, MSF started a nutritional program, including two inpatient centers for severe acute malnutrition. At the same time, a new approach was adopted: after a limited period of hospitalization in a typical nutritional facility, the treatment was then continued at home with weekly medical checkups. According to an MSF assessment, the outpatient treatment was possible with the use of "ready-to-use specialized food" (Priem, 2002). The report specified that "the MSF team was initially a little reluctant to set up this outpatient phase of treatment, essentially because of fear of relapses" (Priem, 2002, p. 11, 20–21). "The teams were worried about not being able to monitor the development of medical complications, as it was difficult for mothers to travel to MSF's facilities. Malnourished children have lower levels of immune defenses."[6] Despite these fears, the new strategy was progressively implemented. In November 2001, in Dakoro, in the Maradi Province, 80% of children initially hospitalized were then transferred to the outpatient phase of treatment (i.e., nutritional rehabilitation at home). Assessment revealed a weakness in the program (a high dropout rate), but nonetheless concluded that home-based nutritional rehabilitation was "satisfactory." The evaluation was based on traditional indicators such as daily mean weight gain, mean duration of treatment, the percentage of readmissions to hospital from home, and the "modes of exit" from the program—cured, defaulted, or deceased.

Steve Collins, a doctor working with Concern, an Irish NGO, had been using ready-to-use foods since 2000, and had demonstrated the effectiveness of home-based care (Collins, 2002). MSF was not then in favor of the strategy, as such limited medical help was deemed too risky for severely malnourished children.

Driven by senior staff convinced of the work by Steve Collins, in July 2003 MSF decided to initiate treatment at home except in complicated cases requiring hospitalization (Tectonidis, 2004). This decision aroused misgivings among MSF medical practitioners. Indeed, many of those working in the field were worried that the positive effect of the home-based treatment might be of shorter duration than that obtained in conven-

6   Quote from an MSF doctor.

tional, inpatient therapeutic feeding centers. Another worry was that mothers would not keep the ready-to-use therapeutic food solely for their malnourished children but share it with all their children (Priem, 2002, p. 20, 22). Defenders of the program responded with field data on the "extensive outpatient phase treatment of malnutrition" (Tectonidis, 2005b), which showed low rates of readmission to hospital, lower relapse rates, and comparable daily mean weight gains overall for the programs. The arguments heard during the outpatient strategy controversy were varied. Defenders of the policy evoked arguments and data from clinical experiences, while its detractors stressed the weaknesses witnessed during the first years of the programs (July 2001 to July 2003) and asked cultural and sociological questions about mothers' behavior: "How can we be sure that they respect treatment regimes once at home?"

MSF Put to the Test by the 2005 Crisis

In February 2005 MSF noticed that admissions to nutritional programs had risen compared with February 2004. This trend was confirmed over the following months. The continuing increase in admissions led to the three press releases mentioned earlier. Senior MSF staff in charge of operations in Niger were initially hesitant to describe the situation as a crisis requiring specific emergency responses, however. Perhaps the rise in the number of admissions was mainly because Nigerien mothers, confronted with chronic poverty-provoking cycles of acute malnutrition, recognized the efficacy of the outpatient programs. Was it MSF's responsibility to respond to an endemic problem linked to poverty? These doubts and questions were raised by some of those in charge.

While disagreement continued within the organization on how to identify signs of danger and the limits of humanitarian responsibility, new indicators and arguments were used publicly to illustrate the gravity of the situation. The results of several nutritional surveys conducted by various institutions, including MSF,[7] were particularly pertinent. Furthermore—and this was the decisive argument within MSF—the need for medical care and the number of admissions to nutritional facilities were continuing to rise. This was universally agreed upon, but disagreement persisted as to the extent of the humanitarian response. From April to June 2005, press releases stated the gravity of the situation and the urgent need to intervene using both types of indicators: epidemiological survey results, and medical observation and data from MSF nutritional centers.

MSF's main demand on June 9, 2005, was for "free food distributions to populations worst affected by malnutrition," leading to the call for "mobilization of donor agencies and of international organizations, such as the WFP and UNICEF." One of the justifications was the observation that the Nigerien government's plan of action—essentially based on selling cereals at moderate prices—was not improving the situation in the most affected rural areas. From March to July, MSF gradually acquired the capacity to target priority zones by cross-referencing data from treatment facilities, nutritional surveys, and socio-economic indicators (Jézéquel, 2005). The organization was thus able to target priority zones hardest hit by acute infanto-juvenile malnutrition.

In the MSF press releases of June 9, June 28, and August 22, the vast numbers of children arriving at feeding centers were cited as proof of the inefficacy of the government response. MSF produced descriptive statements to demonstrate the gravity of the "acute malnutrition epidemic." The medical diagnosis—

---

7   Nutritional and Retroactive Mortality survey, Keita, Dakoro, and Mayayi districts, April 2005 (Epicentre); Food Security survey in the Tahoua district, May 2005 (MSF-France); survey by Helen Keller International and the WFP in the Maradi and Zinder regions in January 2005, revealing "alarming levels of malnutrition" and recognizing that "the situation in these two regions of Niger, and probably other regions, is comparable to those of populations living in war zones or other crises" (WPF, HKI, 2005).

"these are children who will die, and we can save them"—struck a sensitive chord. There were others who shared MSF's point of view. In July 2005 the WFP, breaking with official strategy, began free food distributions. Public controversy flared again, however, sparked by another MSF press release published on August 22, the day before the UN Secretary General was due to arrive in Niger. The press release said the food distributions were insufficient and ill-adapted in terms of geographical targeting. It went on to reproach agencies for not supplying "specialized foods" for very young children who were "dying from hunger" and were the "principal victims of malnutrition." The issue of saving children by providing specialized food was raised repeatedly in public from the end of June (i.e., the beginning of the hunger gap, when the deterioration of the situation had become foreseeable).

This insistence on targeted free food distributions and appropriate solutions for very young children ("from six to fifty-nine months of age") used field experience as a counterargument against the strategies adopted by the Nigerien government and other key institutional actors. MSF's expertise and experience did not explicitly challenge the free market, but described its effects, or rather lack of effects, on the population. In the same vein, MSF requested that all health care for children be free of charge for the duration of the hunger gap.

What were the alternative doctrines and policies to those recommended by MSF and other humanitarian organizations (particularly Action Against Hunger)? On the one hand, there was what could be described as an analytical contention, and, on the other, a more polemical contention during peak moments of controversy.

USAID was quick to offer opposing analytical arguments (USAID, 2005). First, the agency recognized the existence of a "grave nutritional crisis" in certain areas of Niger: a "predictable and inevitable" result of chronic poverty. The authors of the document contested the number of people at risk according to "certain press reports," then affirmed that 2.4 million to 3.6 million people were exposed to food shortages, and that "some will die from lack of food, poor quality water, or other problems not linked to food." This fatalistic judgment did not explicitly target MSF, but challenged the effectiveness of the association's food aid policy, which was not seen to take into account the multi-factorial character of child mortality. The type of aid that MSF provided meant that it responded locally to the emergency, but did not address the factors aggravating malnutrition. The authors believed it was necessary to study these other factors and the food situation in the most affected zones of Niger where MSF was working (alongside many other agencies from July 2005 onwards). In the end, the analysis did not disagree with MSF's activities, as it recommended immediate emergency aid including free food distributions and "food supplements for children less than five years old." But the causes of the crisis were not, and could not, be tackled this way, and there was a lot of skepticism regarding the medical solutions offered by MSF.

One controversy sparked by MSF's interventions began with two BBC reports of September 13 and 15, 2005, about MSF's accusation that the WFP was not delivering aid to those most in need.[8]

On September 15, the WFP's director sent a letter to the president of MSF-France protesting the condemnation of his organization. This was in contrast to the cooperation between the WFP and all MSF sections in the field. He believed that private

8   BBC News, September 13, 2005, and BBC TV, 15 September 15, 2005: Hilary Andersson, "Niger food is 'misdirected.'" The WFP responded (without mentioning the BBC) in a press release published in Niamey on September 15: "More food to the most needy—WFP moves into next phase of Niger operation."

discussions were preferable to public confrontation, as the latter was counterproductive. In other words, progress is not made by denouncing one's partners in the press, but by speaking with them directly; and MSF was not helping malnourished children with its press release, but just gaining publicity. The WFP's director suggested setting up a forum with MSF to discuss operational problems and to come to a "common understanding" of working with the media. In his opinion, there was no split between MSF and the WFP; they should still work together. The president of MSF France responded that public controversy had achieved better results than meetings with aid organizations. The public debate had convinced relief organizations and the Nigerien authorities of the necessity of distributing food, and of giving priority to zones with the highest levels of acute malnutrition, which had not been the case up to mid-July.

In the end, the aid objectives announced by the WFP in its press release September 15, 2005, matched the emergency priorities defined by MSF.

Nutritional Strategies and "Ready-to-Use Therapeutic Foods" (RUTFs)

Ready-to-Use Foods and Prevention

During 2005 the MSF sections in Niger treated sixty thousand children suffering from severe acute malnutrition, adopting the method initiated by Steve Collins in 2000. MSF's innovation was not the method but its application on such a large scale and with such high cure rates (over 80%). This was unprecedented; it was the first time that it had been proven possible to treat such a large number of children with severe acute malnutrition. Over the summer of 2005 the Ministry of Health embraced this strategy in their revised national treatment protocol for severe acute malnutrition.

In 2006 MSF staff in Paris responsible for operations in Niger decided to no longer limit RUTFs to the treatment of severe acute malnutrition, but to use them from the earlier stage of moderate malnutrition. The extended use of RUTFs was initially trialed in two of the hardest-hit districts of the Maradi province in 2006. At the end of the year, all involved agreed on the operation's medical efficacy, but also on its very high cost. The cost was partly due to the price of Plumpy'nut, but more significantly to screenings carried out to identify patients suffering from acute malnutrition. Consequently, the decision was taken to simplify care and to stop selecting children based on whether they were suffering from acute malnutrition or not. During the hunger gap period (May to October), in one district, all children in the age group most in danger (six months to three years of age) would receive a daily nutritional supplement in the form of a new ready-to-use product, Plumpy'doz,[9] while children with severe acute malnutrition would receive specific treatment in a therapeutic program (twenty-two thousand cases in 2007).

During the evaluation of this strategy at the end of 2007, program managers observed that the number of admissions compared with those of preceding years (2002–2005) had dropped from June onwards and stayed relatively low until October. The strategy of general distribution to all children up to three years of age adopted in 2007 had the same effect in terms of the reduction of the number of cases of severe acute malnutrition as the method of selection used in 2006. This information justified the early intervention strategy (i.e., the distribution of Plumpy'doz to all children from six months to three years of age during the six-month period of the year when hunger gaps are recurrent). In terms of budget, detailed analysis

9   Plumpy'doz is a dense, ready-to-use food. Made of milk powder, oil, sugar, and micro nutrients, it is rich in vitamins and minerals. Unlike Plumpy'nut, it is complementary to a child's normal diet. It contains all the vitamins and minerals required for growth, but only some of the proteins and calories.

of spending in the district of Guidam Roumji showed that 77% of the budget was spent on specialized food for children in 2007, comparing favorably with just 35% in 2006, when large-scale selection operations where required. MSF does not generally recommend early distributions of ready-to-use foods to whole age groups for several months a year in all situations of chronic malnutrition, but recommends it in cases of high levels of acute malnutrition and associated mortality.

The above summary of MSF operations in Niger was based on information given to us by their initiators. A reminder of some of the controversies linked to the increased use of ready-to-use foods should also be provided.

In 2007, when the Niger program managers proposed early intervention with the main argument of simplifying treatment, there were strong objections within the association. Some challenged whether such an extension of the program should be MSF's responsibility; they believed that such chronic problems are the domain of development policies and not of emergency organizations such as MSF. They believed that MSF should limit itself to treating epidemics of severe acute malnutrition using the validated outpatient treatment strategies, and avoid extending treatment to prevention in moderately malnourished children or all children in poorer countries. Similar criticisms were expressed by other organizations, accusing MSF of proposing only a medical solution to the problem of under-nourishment, whereas it includes much wider factors. Current emergency medical methods for severe cases cannot be generalized in the long term—to reduce under-nourishment, other factors and constraints must be taken into account: economics, agriculture, sociology, etc. MSF responded that child mortality was catastrophically high in zones with high incidences of under-nourishment, and that a medical means of reducing mortality rates existed. The results obtained in Niger showed that it was possible to reduce severe acute malnutrition in high-risk zones by distributing preventive ready-to-eat foods to all children from six to thirty-six months of age. Why then wait for the children to become severely sick and come for a consultation before proposing treatment?

An article published in *Science* (Enserink, 2008, p. 36) suggested—wrongly according to some (Bradol, 2008)—that MSF advocated a strategy of universal prevention by the distribution of fortified milk paste to millions of under-nourished children in sub-Saharan Africa and South Asia. In 2005, 19.3 million children were estimated to be suffering from severe acute malnutrition worldwide, and another 178 million suffering from stunted growth (Black, 2008, p. 245). Within MSF, it was generally accepted that priority must be given to populations where malnutrition causes high mortality rates or where it is most prevalent. Nonetheless, other than severe epidemic flare-ups, not everyone agreed on intervention thresholds, whether at a population level or for individual patients. As with many controversies within MSF, disagreements on practical intervention strategies were linked to the recurring issue of MSF's role and its medical and humanitarian responsibilities.

The Cost of Ready-to-Use Foods

MSF identified the cost of ready-to-use foods as a problem early in 2002, and support for local production in Niger was considered to help reduce costs. At this point, Plumpy'nut-type milk pastes were limited to the treatment of severe acute malnutrition. The question of cost only really came to the fore after 2006, when MSF advocated wider-scale use of these products.

There was little scientific opposition at the time to the use of ready-to-use milk-based foods for the treatment of moderate acute malnutrition or as preventive dietary supplements in regions where malnutrition was a serious health problem causing high mortality in young children. Because of the cost, however, this kind of strategy was not regarded as realistic, and as such the recommended use of these products was limited to severe cases. It was also stressed that this nutritional strategy would create further economic dependence because of its cost and need for international funding (UNDP, Integrated Regional Information Networks, September 6, 2006).

MSF publicly recognized the economic factor as a problem. It was true that wider-scale use of RUTFs would not be feasible without reducing production costs and increasing funds for nutritional programs.[10] MSF nevertheless maintained that treatment could not be restricted to severely malnourished children when intervening in regions with high incidences of malnutrition, even in the short term. In countries such as Niger, recommending restricted treatment would lead to queues of starving children, huge therapeutic feeding centers, and inevitable media attention. It was understandable that such a poor image of countries in difficulty was not acceptable to their governments.

The Constructive Role of Controversies

This analysis of controversies and public disagreements reveals the conflictual nature of the process of innovation. Cases of malaria and under-nutrition are in no way exceptional, and senior MSF staff members are used to dealing with controversies. It is part of the usual procedure, inseparable from medical care whenever alternative medical practices need to be adopted as the standard. In this document, we have described how MSF deals with such controversies, and what results it has achieved.

10   According to a study published in *The Lancet* (Morris et al., 2008), international funding for malnutrition did not exceed $250–300 million a year for 2000 to 2005. According to the authors, if that sum were distributed in its entirety to the twenty countries with the highest levels of malnutrition, this would only represent two dollars per malnourished child.

MSF treatment protocols regarding ACTs became recognized international recommendations after a period of disagreement. In the treatment of severe acute malnutrition, MSF demonstrated the large-scale feasibility and effectiveness of a strategy set up by several institutions (*Institut de Recherche pour le Développement*, the WHO, universities, Nutriset) and NGOs (Action against Hunger, Concern).[11]

After the 2005 crisis, Nigerien authorities, donor agencies, and international aid agencies adopted several new measures including treatment of severe acute malnutrition at home with new generation foods, treatment of moderate malnutrition with standard cereals, and free medical treatment for children and pregnant women. Unfortunately, apart from centers supported by international organizations, free care for children and pregnant women was not feasible due to lack of funds.

The number of children treated for malnutrition in Niger increased from a few thousand before 2005 to more than three hundred thousand in 2006. But the move towards a medical intervention aimed at reducing the incidence of severe acute malnutrition through early distribution of nutritious foods still attracts criticisms and questions. Local results have not been sufficient to justify implementing these strategies or to end disagreements about the need for epidemiological proof of effectiveness. This is why MSF is launching a debate on the economic and political dogmas used to restrict nutritional programs.

---

11   In June 2007 several UN organisations, including the WHO, announced that they recommended home-based care and the distribution of RUTFs as treatment protocols for uncomplicated severe acute malnutrition (WHO, WFP, UNICEF, 2007).

Bibliography

Black, R., L. Allen, Z. Bhutta, L. Caulfield, M. De Onis, M. Ezzati, C. Mathers, J. Rivera; Maternal and Child Undernutrition Study Group. 2008. "Maternal and child undernutrition: global and regional exposures and health consequences." *The Lancet* 371 (9608): 243–260.

Bradol, J.-H. 2007. "Niger 2005: l'année du biscuit." *In Niger 2005. Une catastrophe si naturelle*, X. Crombé, J.-H. Jézéquel, editors. 273–294. Paris, Karthala: MSF.

——. 2008. "Responses to a seasonal high incidence of severe acute malnutrition, operational lessons and policy changes." Symposium at "Starved for Attention. The Neglected Crisis of Childhood Malnutrition," Columbia University, New York, September 11–12.

Collins, S. 2002. "Outpatient care for severely malnourished children in emergency relief programmes: a retrospective cohort study." *The Lancet* 360 (9348): 1824–1830.

Crombé, X., J.-H. Jézéquel, editors. 2007. *Niger 2005. Une catastrophe si naturelle*. Paris, Karthala: MSF.

Enserink, M. 2008. "The Peanut Butter Debate." *Science* 322: 36–38.

Gastellu-Etchegorry, M., F. Matthys, M. Galinski, N. J. White, F. Nosten. 2001. "Malaria epidemic in Burundi." *The Lancet* 357 (9261): 1046–1047.

Guthmann, J.-P., M. Bonnet, L. Ahoua, F. Dantoine, S. Balkan. 2007. "Death Rates from Malaria Epidemics, Burundi and Ethiopia." *Emerging Infectious Diseases* 13 (1): 140–143.

Guthmann, J.-P., F. Checchi, I. Van den Broek, S. Balkan, M. Van Herp, E. Comte, O. Bernal, J-M Kindermans, S. Venis, D. Legros, P. Guerin. 2008. "Assessing Antimalarial Efficacy in a Time of Change to Artemisinin-Based Combination Therapies: The Role of Médecins Sans Frontières." *PloS Medicine* 5 (8): 1191–1199.

Jézéquel, J.-H. 2005. *"Ici, l'enfant n'a pas de valeur"*. *Sécurité alimentaire, malnutrition et développement au Niger.* Paris: Médecins Sans Frontières.

Kassankogno, Y., R. Allan, C. Delacollette. 2000. *Management of malaria in epidemic affected areas of Burundi.* Geneva: World Health Organization.

Lemieux, C. 2007. "A quoi sert l'analyse des controverses?" *Mil neuf cent, revue d'histoire intellectuelle* 25: 191–212.

Morris, S., B. Cogill, R. Uauy. 2008. "Effective international action against undernutrition: why has it proven so difficult and what can be done to accelerate progress?" *The Lancet* 371 (9612): 608–621.

Nosten, F., M. Van Vugt, C. Luxemburger, K.L. Thway, A. Brockman, R. McGready. F. Ter Kuile, S. Looareesuwan, N.J. White. "Effects of artesunate-mefloquine combination on incidence of Plasmodium falciparum malaria and mefloquine resistance in western Thailand: a prospective study." *The Lancet* 356 (9226): 297–302.

Olivier de Sardan, J.-P. 2008. "Introduction thématique. La crise alimentaire de 2004–2005 au Niger en contexte." *Afrique contemporaine* 225: 17–37.

Packard, R. M. 2007. *The Making of a Tropical Disease. A Short History of Malaria.* Baltimore, The Johns Hopkins University Press.

Priem, V. 2002. *Évaluation de l'intervention médico-nutritionnelle de Médecins Sans Frontières sur le département de Maradi. Missions Dakoro et Maradi. Août 2001-janvier 2002. Niger.* Paris: Médecins Sans Frontières.

Tectonidis, M. 2004. *MSF au Niger. Projet nutritionnel de Maradi. Visite du 8 au 19 mars 2004,* MSF archives, Paris.

——. 2005a. *Historique et analyse du programme de nutrition de Maradi.* MSF archives, Paris.

——. 2005b. *Prise en charge ambulatoire de la malnutrition aiguë.* MSF archives, Paris.

——. 2006. "Crisis in Niger—Outpatient Care for Severe Acute Malnutrition." *New England Journal of Medicine* 354: 224–227.

United States Agency for International Development (USAID). 2005. *Niger: An Evidence Base For Understanding The Current Crisis (28 July 2005).* Washington: United States Agency for International Development.

World Health Organization (WHO). 2001. *Antimalarial Drug Combination Therapy: Report of a WHO Informal Consultation.* Geneva: World Health Organization.

——. 2007. *Community-based management of severe acute malnutrition. A Joint Statement by the World Health Organization, the World Food Programme, the United Nations System Standing Committee on Nutrition and the United Nations Children's Fund.* Geneva, Rome, New York: World Health Organization, Standing Committee on Nutrition, World Food Programme, United Nations Children's Fund.

World Food Programme (WFP), Helen Keller International (HKI). 2005. *Évaluation de base de l'état nutritionnel des enfants de 6 à 59 mois dans les régions rurales de Maradi et de Zinder. Rapport de deux enquêtes.* Niamey: World Food Programme, Helen Keller International.

World Food Programme. 2006. *Annual Report 2005.* Rome: World Food Programme.

Chapter 5

Cholera

Diagnosis and Treatment Outside the Hospital

Jean-François Corty

Cholera spread from Asia during the nineteenth century in successive waves of epidemics. Several pandemics extended from the Middle East following commercial trading routes, troop movements, and pilgrimages. The reduction in transport times and the increase in population movements contributed to the spread of the disease (Bourdelais and Dodin, 1987, p. 33). Mecca, which is a focal point for pilgrims from all continents, became a hub for *Vibrio cholerae* O1. The disease seemed under control at the beginning of the twentieth century, thanks mainly to improvements in hygiene and water management in large industrial cities. Nothing foretold the emergence of a seventh pandemic in 1961, which was just as lethal as the six preceding identified periods of transmission and is still active today. From the departure point in the Sulawesi Islands, cholera spread through the Far East, arriving in the 1970s in Western Europe through Spain, and Africa through Guinea. Following the Niger River, the disease affected neighboring African countries and spread across the continent.

The pandemic involved a new strain of the cholera bacteria, named El Tor, discovered in 1905 in a lazaretto (quarantine station) of the same name in Mecca. A biotype of the O1 strain, it is found today on all continents, replacing the previously dominant O1 classic biotype. Following an epidemic outbreak in Peru in the early 1990s, the pandemic spread through South

88

America, which had previously been spared.

Cholera is currently present in almost fifty countries. Africa is the most affected continent and accounts for 95% of all reported cases, followed by Asia, and, to a lesser extent, the Americas, Europe, and Oceania, the latter two reporting almost uniquely imported cases. In 2005, 131,943 cases were reported worldwide, including 2,272 deaths, a specific mortality rate[1] of 1.72%. Real numbers are thought to be much higher; it is estimated that only 5% to 10% of all cases are actually reported, and that there are other shortcomings with surveillance systems (World Health Organization [WHO], 2006). A strain belonging to a new serogroup, *Vibrio cholerae* O139, appeared in the Gulf of Bengal in 1992 and has remained localized in Asia for the time being (WHO, 1996; WHO, 2004b).

Robert Koch identified the *Vibrio cholerae* O1 bacillus in 1883, beating Pasteur, whose research methods were based on the study of immunity mechanisms rather than on identifying the causal agent. During epidemics, direct inter-human transmission is the most frequent mode of infection, whether it be from a sick patient, a healthy carrier, an infected cadaver, or from feces-contaminated drinking water or food. In non-epidemic periods, aquatic plants, crustaceans, and mollusks are the reservoirs for the bacteria. These are environments where it can survive indefinitely under the right conditions. Clinical features of the disease mainly include profuse watery stools, sometimes associated with vomiting, and subsequent rapid dehydration. The natural course of the disease leads to death in 50% of symptomatic cases. Survivors may recover in four to six days, with an acquired immunity after one week, which might last several months. The main treatment is rehydration, either orally or by intravenous infusion, depending on the clinical state. Antibiotic therapy is sometimes used. The treatment is well

---

1   Specific mortality rate: the ratio of the number of deaths due to a certain disease over the number of new cases during a defined time period.

known and has an undeniable effect on mortality, but mortality remains high in countries where health systems are not mobilized when faced with epidemics.

Research progresses slowly, and a useful vaccine[2] has yet to be found for this disease that essentially affects poor populations.

The Cholera Camp, a Curative Innovation Based on New Organizational and Logistical Set-ups

Creation, Objectives, and Organization of the Cholera Camp

Cholera spread throughout Africa in the 1980s. MSF intervened regularly in refugee and displaced persons camps, known as "closed settings,"[3] which were favorable to cholera propagation. Such was the case in Korem, Ethiopia; the Ethiopian refugee camp in Wad Kaoli, Sudan in 1985; and in 1988 in Malawi in the Mankhokwe Mozambican refugee camp. Then, from 1988 to 1993, again in Malawi, a series of epidemics affected other Mozambican refugee camps, where over seven thousand cases were treated. From July to August 1994, during the mass grouping of Rwandan refugees in East Zaire, a major epidemic occurred, with fifty-eight thousand cases and 4,200 deaths. Here the specific mortality rate reached 22% in the first three days (Brown et al., 2002; Goma Epidemiology Group, 1995).

In March 1985, MSF had been assisting a displaced population of around forty thousand people in Korem, North Wolo Province, Ethiopia, for over a year. Living conditions were deplorable: plastic sheets for shelter and no blankets despite night temperatures approaching zero. One of the doctors remembers a group of corrugated barracks acting as a hospital where around seven

---

2   Despite the efforts of certain organizations—such as the International Vaccine Institute—that are fighting to develop a vaccine.

3   Closed settings are delimited geographical areas in which population figures are known, whereas in open settings, whether urban or rural, indicators are more difficult to quantify because of distances and population movements, etc.

hundred patients were treated. The average weight of hospitalized adults was thirty-three kilograms. It was in these conditions that almost two thousand people were hit by a cholera epidemic lasting over two months—an attack rate[4] of nearly 5%, common in this kind of setting where crowding, hygiene, and the weakened state of the people favor disease transmission in general. The MSF teams, inexperienced in this type of situation, tried to organize a tent isolation camp to treat sick patients. They set up the necessary sanitation systems to prevent the spread of disease (i.e., water-source protection), and systematically carried out identification of sick patients in family shelters. The WHO recommended mass prophylaxis treatment with a long-acting, single-dose sulphamide, Fansadil, which was distributed by the teams. Neither the WHO, the Centers for Disease Control and Prevention (CDC), nor MSF was certain as to the effectiveness of this treatment.

This experience presented the teams with the organizational challenges of caring for a high number of patients over a short period of time. The medical protocols were simple but unwieldy;[5] fifty to one hundred patients could be receiving intravenous treatment at any one time, assuming sufficient medical supplies.

These initial operational strategies in response to closed-setting epidemics were then applied in Malawi. Between 1986 and 1988, around four hundred thousand Mozambican refugees settled in villages and camps along the border. There were a total of nine hundred thousand refugees in Malawi by 1990. MSF had been providing medical care in the south of the country since 1986, and, in March 1988, the first cases of the epidemic occurred in the Mankhokwe camp, with a population of nearly thirty thousand people. The epidemic continued until May, and

---

4   Attack rate: the number of cumulated cases as a percentage of a given population over a defined period.

5   The protocols required large quantities of intravenous fluid treatment, and constant and meticulous vital signs surveillance.

951 cases were treated by MSF in collaboration with Mozambican medical staff and the Malawian authorities. Response strategy included identifying the cases, and patient care in a cholera treatment center (CTC), or cholera camp. Preventive measures were also employed, including market and public site closures, contact prophylaxis,[6] and water chlorination (MSF, 1988). The first field involvement of Epicentre, in 1988, also showed the relevance of improving coordination of epidemiology and emergency medical action.

The creation of the CTC model remains MSF's most significant contribution to cholera epidemic response. Patient care and epidemiology were the two priorities, and the CTC provides rapid medical care to a large number of patients while isolating them from hospital structures where disease may spread. This strategy requires significant logistical resources so that medical care, treatment and recovery, as well as shelter, food, and water supply are all provided in simple, functional, and autonomous conditions.

In practice, isolation, supply, and hygiene were the three key elements of a functional CTC, and opening a structure was indicated once more than five new cases per day are identified in a closed setting such as a camp, a prison, or a social or sanitary institution (MSF, 1995). In terms of isolation, the cholera camp is closed and different from other care structures. It includes four separate entities, so as to regulate patient and caregiver movement, thus limiting the risk of transmission. One unit acts as a triage and observation center for suspected cases, another for hospitalization or isolation, including disinfection measures. A convalescence unit treats patients receiving oral rehydration therapy. Finally, the "neutral" zone houses the kitchen, supplies, and changing rooms. In terms of supplies, the center must be able to maintain sufficient medical and non-medical stocks

---

6   Contact prophylaxis consists of preventive antibiotic treatments for people in contact with a patient.

to provide care (for cholera, but also for common associated diseases such as malaria, etc.), as well as lodging and food for all patients, to which must be added sixty liters of water per day per person[7] to guarantee the center's autonomy. The teams use tools developed by MSF, Epicentre, and MSF-Logistique to plan cholera center management and supplies, notably the cholera guide and cholera kits. Furthermore, in bigger camps, oral rehydration units are created in the periphery so as to begin treatment immediately, before transfer to the CTC, if indicated.

MSF thus developed emergency cholera response expertise from 1985 to 1989 in smaller camps. In the 1990s this knowledge was developed to use on a completely different scale, for epidemics in camps containing hundreds of thousands of people. These methods are still in use and pertinent today.

Medical Practice in the CTC

Two major controversies concerning medical protocols within CTCs have stimulated debate among specialists. The first involves intravenous fluid rehydration. Since the middle of the twentieth century, it has been common practice to rapidly administer large volumes of intravenous fluids to treat severe cases. This practice is not without complications, however (hypoglycemia, pulmonary edema in older patients and children, and hypokalemia), and was only administered in hospitals or health centers, whereas CTCs are deliberately created outside existing hospital structures. At the same time, a process of active case-finding in closed settings replaced passively waiting for patients to turn up. To achieve this, clinicians accustomed to hospital settings and uncomfortable with these new strategies were sometimes given specific training. Around this time, however, the WHO and the United Nations Children's Fund (UNICEF) questioned the use of large-volume intravenous rehydration strategies and recom-

---

7   MSF worked on the availability and use of granulated chlorine, establishing varying standardized dilutions depending on intended use, from drinking water through to disinfection.

mended oral rehydration, which in part explained the differences between the WHO and MSF cholera kits.

The second controversy concerned doxycycline. According the WHO, the cholera bacillus is commonly resistant to this drug, and prophylaxis only recommended for contacts of sick patients where at least one secondary case has occurred in a family of five. Despite this, doxycycline is still part of the MSF and WHO cholera kit. In an article in 2002, MSF detailed the limits of antibiotic therapy: "Antibiotic use is only envisaged for the most severe cases. It is useful for reducing diarrhea duration and volume, and germ carriage time" (Brown et al., 2002). The same article restated the absolute priority of rehydration: "Deaths in cholera camps are essentially due to delays in quality rehydration treatment: if this treatment is applied rigorously, specific mortality drops to less than 0.5% (in refugee camps). Standardizing antibiotic therapy risks inducing a false sense of security in medical staff and distracting from essential rehydration. ... Preventive antibiotics may be recommended in cholera epidemics affecting populations in closed settings (e.g., prisons)."[8] So MSF did not recommend curative antibiotic treatment during cholera epidemics—with exceptions for severe cases and situations of very high population density.

Cholera Guides and Kits: Tools for Emergency Responses

The idea of a kit for immediate responses during cholera epidemics was proposed a few weeks after the disastrous situation and shortages in Korem in 1985. Cholera cases cause concern, which may sometimes lead to importation problems.[9] That's why the cholera kit was called the "001 kit," because cholera was the first disease on the WHO obligatory declared diseases list. The kit is designed for around six hundred patients and essentially includes intravenous material (Ringer's Lactate),

---

8 *Journée en hommage à Lapeyssonnie*, Le Pharo, Marseille, 20 March 2002.

9 National authorities sometimes refuse officially to declare cholera epidemics for various political reasons.

oral rehydration salts in sachets, an antibiotic (doxycycline), and chlorination material. With this kit, MSF contributed to the standardization of Ringer's Lactate, and the large quantities provided avoid stock shortages of this essential item.

The kit contents caused and still cause controversy involving MSF and the WHO. MSF teams working with epidemics aim first to treat the severest cases. The WHO approaches cholera from a more theoretical angle, based notably on epidemic response strategies developed by the Bangladesh International Center for Diarrhoeal Disease Research (ICDDR), which predict an attack rate of 0.2% for the entire population during epidemic outbreaks in an open setting, of which around 20% are severe. MSF's experience in Mozambican refugee camps in Malawi showed attack rates of 1% to 2% or higher. Differences in opinions resulted in an MSF kit which contains 80% intravenous treatments and 20% oral, and a WHO kit with contents of inverse proportions (Bitar, 1991b). To adapt to open-setting epidemics affecting populations spread over large areas, the 001 kit may be split into mini-kits, each treating twenty severe cases, for smaller peripheral treatment centers.

The first reference document was written by field teams in 1980 to provide clear and practical objectives for cholera epidemic response (MSF, 1980). The first guide recounting MSF experiences in closed settings was published in 1995, and stresses the cholera camp model, rehydration protocols, and water chlorination. Revision of the guide began in 1997, and was completed in 2004. The revised guide included strategies for epidemic control in open settings.

The WHO published *Guidelines for Cholera Control* in 1993. While there are no references to MSF publications or associated authors (WHO, 1993), it nevertheless includes the cholera camp model, which is used as a reference by many health actors.

Curative Care in Open Settings

MSF-Belgium and MSF-Holland were already present in Peru when the seventh cholera pandemic struck the continent in the early 1990s. In 1991, at the height of the epidemic, five operational sections developed a common response mission (Belgium, France, Holland, Switzerland, and Spain). Within three months of the arrival of the cholera bacillus on the continent, the WHO created the Global Task Force on Cholera Control, with the main objectives of promoting disease control and research and development initiatives. At the same time, MSF opened an international emergency response base in Central America, initially in El Salvador, then in Costa Rica, which eventually closed in 2000. The base offered technical and training support in cholera epidemic responses for both MSF teams and regional medical staff.

Lima, with a population of seven million, was struck by the disease, but quickly benefited from national and international humanitarian organizations that used their previous experience in urban settings. MSF then decided to intervene in peripheral rural areas where help was harder to obtain: first on the coast, then in the mountains, and finally in the jungle. These interventions involved eight provinces and continued for over a year.

Epidemic control in these contexts required new operational strategies.[10] The purely medical aspects had been defined and would not change (rehydration and antibiotic protocols). Moreover, no effective vaccine then existed for prevention, nor were there any rapid diagnostic tests available. The changes made were in the organization of preventive and curative care.

Affected populations were spread out and difficult to access in mountainous and jungle zones, so large CTCs could not cater to needs. The objective was to get as close to affected popu-

---

10   At the beginning of the 1990s the Shining Path was very active, particularly in the capital, so epidemic control was carried out in a violent context.

lations as possible, using existing structures. Care was decentralized to mini-CTCs known as cholera treatment units and oral rehydration solution (ORS) points, supported by mobile teams. These structures were associated with official health centers, and on-site personnel were trained in cholera care and received appropriate supplies. Each center had a capacity to treat four to five severe cases at any one time. Supply and supervision were provided by regular visits that also served to update epidemiological data. MSF used the UNICEF child diarrhea rehydration program, an existing network from which operations for the population as a whole could be developed.

Peru was MSF's first large-scale, open rural setting cholera mission.[11] In the 1990s, following several similar interventions and in-house reflection on how to adapt response strategies, Epicentre published a report setting out the first recommendations for these kinds of epidemics (Dorlencourt, 1997). It specified that an initial, thorough, pluridisciplinary evaluation (exploratory mission) was necessary to develop responses. The report also stressed that the epidemic must officially be declared by health authorities conforming to WHO definitions, that initial suspect cases must be confirmed in reference laboratories, but also that the medical and sanitary context must be evaluated before deciding upon an appropriate intervention strategy. Clinical patient care must be carried out and documented using patient treatment cards from cholera kits.

It is also necessary to advertise that health care is free of cost, with the help of local authorities. The recommendations also insisted upon the necessity of establishing a simple functional surveillance system in treatment centers, ORS points, and health structures in the intervention zone.

---

11   Urban operations involving mobile teams were developed by MSF-Belgium during epidemics in Guinea and Liberia in 1990 and 1991 (Wuillaume, 1992).

The cholera camp model remains MSF's major contribution in terms of organizational, logistical, and curative innovation. Its clear effect on mortality inside but also outside camps has been recognized, and the model reproduced.

Other Measures Associated with Curative Care

Coupling of Epidemiology and Emergency Medical Action

In 1988, MSF associated an epidemiological survey with curative care during the cholera epidemic affecting Mozambican refugees. Epicentre conducted an investigation aimed at describing epidemic characteristics regarding timing, locations, and people affected, to better define epidemic breadth, severity, and evolution. This also allowed the definition of more appropriate curative response strategies, the modification of actions where needed, the identification of potential risk factors, and the development of recommendations aiming to reduce epidemic spread (Moren, Stefanaggi, Antona, et al., 1991).

In general, this kind of survey is based on a simple field-data collection system, involving the location, date, number of cases, their age distribution, and number of deaths. These parameters allow the calculation of the main epidemic surveillance indicators, which are attack rates and case fatality rates. These data are collected by health agents locally and by sections heads in displaced persons camps, but also in health structures and in cemetery surveys.

Several Epicentre reports summarize MSF's care experience in a dozen epidemics, notably in Malawi and in Peru (Bitar, 1991a, 1991b; Wuillaume, 1992; Dorlencourt, 1997).

In short, cholera epidemic control measures in refugee camps were and still are technically simple and easy to master, and well supported by guides and kits produced by MSF. These measures also aimed to demonstrate the possibility of reducing mortality rates to less than 0.5% in closed settings thanks to CTCs. MSF has achieved this result not just once but repeatedly.

Furthermore, interventions in refugee camps have led to the analysis of closed-setting epidemics. The dramatic increase in the number of cases reaches a peak in a short time period, mostly within two to four weeks. The epidemic rarely lasts more than a few weeks, probably because of population density, whereas the average duration of open-setting epidemics is four to five months. Closed-setting attack rates are usually higher than in open settings, and may reach or exceed 5% (Brown et al., 2002).

Epidemiological monitoring in open settings developed from indicators used in refugee camps. The monitoring established in Peru aimed to anticipate epidemic evolution using a classical database, contamination sources, and new-case mapping, but also led to uncertainty due to the difficulties in defining populations moving freely over geographical areas with unclear boundaries. We must therefore remain very cautious if we are confidently to predict a cholera epidemic and its development, and many examples exist as reminders of how epidemic cycles are poorly explained and hard to control.

What distinguishes MSF from other medical actors today is its capacity to mount standardized medical practices and surveillance systems (cases and deaths) in a very short space of time, at scale and with or without the support of epidemiologists.

Diagnosis and Prevention

Diagnostic Tools

MSF participated in the development of rapid diagnostic tests, and MSF and Epicentre both took part in their field validation. The Pasteur Institute developed a rapid test for O1 and O139 *Vibrio cholerae* strains (the One-step Immuno-chromatographic Dipstick) starting in 2000, and performed an initial validation study in 2002 in collaboration with the International Centre for Diarrhoeal Disease Research, Bangladesh (ICDDR,B)[12] in Dhaka. Results were encouraging in endemic situations (Nato et al., 2003). In 2003, the CDC launched a study with the ICDDR and the Pasteur Institute to examine the precision and feasibility of use of three rapid cholera detection tests (SMART, Medicos, and the Pasteur Institute tests). Results showed that the Pasteur Institute test was the most appropriate for detection of the O1 strain in areas where health personnel skills were limited (Kalluri et al., 2006). Another study performed in 2004 by various partners, including MSF, confirmed the performance of the Pasteur Institute test in epidemic field conditions. A new format for this test (one stick with bands for O1 and O139 strains) was validated in the field by Epicentre (Alberti, 2007; Page, Alberti, 2008).

In addition to rapid tests, the cholera strain must be confirmed by a specialized laboratory, often in another country; correct sample-taking and transport conditions must be observed. MSF uses the filter paper transport medium developed in collaboration with the Pasteur Institute, but its efficacy has not yet been proven. Epicentre performed a study comparing filter paper disks, then limited to certain laboratories, to the reference transport medium, Cary-Blair (Page, Alberti, 2008). The question is of increasing importance in current contexts, where there is evidence of antibiotic resistance and new strains, so it is essential that samples arrive safely at reference laboratories.

Vaccination

The effect of cholera vaccination on prevention is still the subject of controversy. The parenteral vaccine developed at the beginning of the twentieth century has not been shown to

---

12   ICDDR,B is one of the main cholera research institutions, collaborating with the WHO.

be effective in prevention, as induced immunity is partial and short-lived (Mosley, Aziz, et al., 1972). In 1973, following a resolution at the Twenty-sixth World Health Assembly, the WHO no longer recommended vaccination for cholera epidemic control (WHO, 1992).

MSF and Epicentre participated in several studies of oral cholera vaccines in the 1990s and early 2000s (Legros, Paquet, Perea, et al., 1999; Epicentre, 1998a; Paquet, 1999; Dorlencourt, Legros, Paquet, 2000; Epicentre, 1998b; Naficy, Rao, Paquet, et al., 1998). In 1999, the WHO concluded in agreement with MSF that vaccinating with the oral bivalent killed whole-cell bacteria vaccine associated with recombinant toxin B subunit (B-Subunit-Whole Cell, or BS-WC, and rBS-WC) was useful in some specific emergency situations, such as refugee camps or high-density slums (WHO, 1999).

In 2001, a senior WHO staff member published an article confirming the importance of vaccination in the prevention of epidemics, in addition to other traditional preventive measures. The author also underlined the importance of further studies to refine vaccination criteria and identify very high-risk populations that might benefit from preventive mass vaccination campaigns (Chaignat, 2001).

The efficacy of the killed whole-cell vaccine with B subunit has been proven (WHO, 2004a), but with just 70% protection over one year; given the efforts required for mass vaccination, its usefulness is limited.

As for preventive vaccination of populations, MSF has participated in working groups to help identify situations in which vaccination would be a valid option in the interest of public health.

Water, Hygiene, and Sanitation

During the epidemic in the Chifunga camp in Malawi in 1990, MSF and Epicentre recommended extending therapeutic care to include prevention (Bitar, Brodel, Gastellu-Etchegorry, et al., 1992).

Evaluations showed the benefits of health education, which means providing clean water and soap to prevent cholera and other hygiene-related illnesses, such as simple and bloody diarrheas and skin and eye diseases, in the camp. Water risk prevention includes bucket chlorination and the banning of suspect water sources. Good water and sanitation programs also avoid contamination of the water table by excreta. Furthermore, all public meeting places were carefully checked or temporarily closed. Finally, corpses were sprinkled with chlorine (orifices in particular) before being enclosed in sealed sacks and buried.

The value of preventive measures remains controversial. For some, the effect is often taken for granted, when in fact it has been only partially proven. Subjective belief in the benefits of prevention overrides the fact-based approach.

Although the effect of clean water supplies on cholera-related mortality is recognized, and targeted actions such as water chlorination and water trucking have been shown to be effective in certain settings, questions remain about the effects of these actions on epidemic occurrence and evolution (Fewtrell et al., 2005). Eradication of the disease in industrialized societies is certainly due to improvements in water supply and hygiene, but also demonstrates the fundamental role of economic, sanitary, and social developments, which cannot be replaced by isolated preventive measures. As for health education in epidemic contexts, effects are doubtful, and benefits unproven.[13]

---

13   MSF-Belgium experiments in the area of cholera epidemic prevention cf. "Water, hygiene and sanitation activities for cholera prevention in communities living adjacent to lake Kivu or Rusizi river, Cyangugu province, Rwanda," communication presented during the cholera conference organised by the WHO and UNICEF, Dakar, 2008.

MSF observed that the hospital-based model of treatment of cholera epidemics was poorly adapted to field situations due to the inability to accept large numbers of patients in acceptable conditions of hygiene. The organization developed a new curative care model, the cholera camp, which has had a proven effect on mortality.

The example of cholera epidemic response in confined areas (camps, prisons) illustrates the creative potential of humanitarian medicine when confronted by the inapplicability of classical treatments in precarious field circumstances. Unfortunately, the majority of all cholera-related deaths occur outside the closed universes described above, and the challenge remains to develop vaccines and other original approaches applicable to the majority of patients.

Bibliography

Alberti, K. 2007. *Validation of a rapid diagnostic test for cholera. Evaluation in field conditions. Study protocol.* Paris: Epicentre, Médecins Sans Frontières.

Bitar, D. 1991a. *Surveillance épidémiologique du choléra dans les missions MSF au Pérou.* Unpublished report. Paris: Epicentre.

——. 1991b. *Surveillance du choléra parmi les réfugiés mozambicains au Malawi, 1988–1991.* Unpublished report. Paris: Epicentre.

Bitar, D., A. Brodel, M. Gastellu-Etchegorry et al. 1992. "Une épidémie de choléra dans un camp de réfugiés mozambicains au Malawi, janvier–février 1990." *Santé Publique* 2: 33–39.

Bourdelais, P., A. Dodin. 1987. *Visages du cholera*. Paris: Éditions Belin.

Brown, V., G. Jacquier, C. Bachy, D. Bitar, D. Legros. "Prise en charge des épidémies de choléra dans un camp de réfugiés." *Bulletin de la Société de Pathologie Exotique*. 95 (5): 351–354.

Chaignat, L. C., 2001. "La place des vaccins dans la lutte contre le cholera." *Médecine Tropicale*. 61: 249-50.

Dorlencourt, F. 1997. *Prise en charge par MSF des épidémies de choléra en milieu ouvert. Revue des 7 dernières années*. Paris: Epicentre.

Dorlencourt, F., D. Legros, C. Paquet. 2000. "Efficacité de la vaccination de masse par deux doses de vaccin anticholérique au cours d'une épidémie dans le district d'Adjumani, en Ouganda." *Bulletin de l'OMS* 2: 209–210.

Epicentre. 1998a. *Use of a two-dose oral cholera vaccine in refugee and displaced populations. Report on a feasibility study conducted in Uganda*. Unpublished report. Paris: Epicentre.

——. 1998b. *Field effectiveness of WC/rBS cholera vaccine during an epidemic in the refugee population of Adjumani district, Uganda*. Unpublished report. Paris: Epicentre.

Fewtrell, L., R. Kaufmann, D. Kay, W. Enanoria, L. Haller, J. Colford, 2005. "Water, sanitation, and hygiene interventions to reduce diarrhoea in less developed countries: a systematic review and meta-analysis." *The Lancet Infectious Diseases* 5 (1): 42–52.

Goma Epidemiology Group. 1995. "Public health impact of Rwandan refugee crisis: what happened in Goma, Zaire, in July, 1994?" *The Lancet* 345 (8946): 339–344.

Kalluri, P., A. Naheed, S. Rahman, M. Ansaruzzaman, A.S. Faruque, M. Bird, F. Khatun, N.A. Bhuiyan, F. Nato, J.M. Fournier, C. Bopp, R.F. Breiman, G.B. Nair, E.D. Mintz. 2006. "Evaluation of three rapid diagnostic tests for cholera: does the skill level of the technician matter?" *Tropical Medicine & International Health* 11 (1): 49–55.

Lapeyssonnie, L. 1971. "Acquisitions récentes en matière d'épidémiologie et de prophylaxie du choléra en Afrique." *Bulletin de la Société de Pathologie Exotique* 64: 644–652.

Legros, D., C. Paquet, W. Perea, I Marty, N.K. Mugisha, H. Royer, M. Neira, B. Ivanhoff. 1999. "Mass vaccination with a two-dose oral cholera vaccine in a refugee camp." *Bulletin WHO* 77 (10): 837842.

Médecins Sans Frontieres (MSF). 1980. *Guide pratique: prise en charge d'une épidémie de choléra dans les camps de réfugiés.* Paris: Médecins Sans Frontieres.

——. 1988. *Le choléra au Malawi.* Unpublished report. Paris: Médecins Sans Frontieres.

——. 1995. *Guide pratique: prise en charge d'une épidémie de choléra*, 1st edition. Paris: Médecins Sans Frontieres.

Moren, A., S. Stefanaggi, D. Antona, D. Bitar, M.G. Etchegorry, M. Tchatchioka, G. Lungu. 1991. "Practical field epidemiology to investigate a cholera outbreak in a Mozambican refugee camp in Malawi, 1988." *Journal of Tropical Medicine and Hygiene* 94: 1–7.

Mosley, W. H., K.M.A. Aziz, A.S.M. Mizanur Rahman, A.K.M. Alauddin Chowdhury, Ansaruddin Ahmen, M. Fahimuddin. 1972. "Report of the 1966–67 cholera vaccine trial in rural East Pakistan. Five years of observation with a practical assessment of the role of a cholera vaccine in cholera control programmes." *Bulletin WHO* 47 (2): 229–238.

Naficy, A., M. R. Rao, C. Paquet, D. Antona, A. Sorkin, J.D. Clemens. 1998. "Treatment and vaccination strategies to control cholera in sub-Saharian refugee settings: a cost-effectiveness analysis." *Journal of the American Medical Association* 279: 521–525.

Nato, F., A. Boutonnier, M. Rajerison, P. Grosjean, S. Darteville, A. Guenole, N.A. Bhuiyan, D.A. Sack, G.B. Nair, J.M. Fournier, S. Chanteau. 2003. "One-Step Immunochromatographic Dipstick Tests for Rapid Detection of Vibrio cholerae O1 and O139 in

Stool Samples." *Clinical and Diagnostic Laboratory Immunology* 10 (3): 476–478.

Page, A.-L., K. Alberti. 2008. *Évaluation d'un test rapide pour le diagnostic du choléra en conditions de terrain pendant une épidémie. Lubumbashi, République Démocratique du Congo.* Paris: Epicentre, Médecins Sans Frontieres.

Paquet, C. 1999. "Vaccination in emergencies." *Vaccine* 17 (3): 116–119.

World Health Organization (WHO). 1992. *Global Task Force on Cholera Control. Guidelines for cholera control*, WHO/CDD/SER/80.4 rev4. Geneva: World Health Organization.

——. 1993. *Guide pour la lutte contre le choléra.* Geneva: World Health Organization.

——. 1996. "Cholera, 1995." *Weekly Epidemiological Record.* 71: 157–164

——. 1999. *Potential use of oral cholera vaccines in emergency situations. Report of a WHO meeting, Geneva, Switzerland, 12–13 May.* WHO/CDS/CSR/EDC/99.4.

——. 2004a. *Cholera vaccines: a new public health tool? Report, WHO meeting, 10–11 December 2002.* Geneva: World Health Organization, Global Task Force on Cholera Control.

——. 2004b. "Cholera, 2003." *Weekly Epidemiological Record* 79 (31): 281–288.

——. 2006. "Cholera, 2005." *Weekly Epidemiological Record* 81 (31): 297–308.

Wuillaume, F. 1992. *Synthèse des activités de lutte contre le choléra développées par MSF-Belgique, 1989–1991.* Unpublished report. Brussels: Médecins Sans Frontières.

Chapter 6

Meningitis

From Practitioner to Prescriber

Eugénie d'Alessandro

Meningococcal cerebrospinal meningitis is caused by a gram-negative diplococcus, *Neisseria meningitidis*, also known as the meningococcus. Although meningococci are present throughout the world, causing sporadic cases and small epidemics, meningococcal disease is a different entity in semi-arid sub-Saharan Africa, where devastating and unpredictable epidemics occur. This phenomenon was first described in the 1960s by Dr. Lapeyssonnie, a French Army general in the medical services. Covering a "band of terrain from the Atlantic to the Red Sea," the meningitis belt is an endemic–epidemic region. The epidemic risk is particularly high during the dry season. The severe consequences of these outbreaks in terms of morbidity and mortality make the disease a public health priority.

Lapeyssonnie refined the first single-dose treatment for meningococcal meningitis epidemics in the early 1960s. His works on the meningococcus and its sensitivity to antibiotic treatment created the hope that "the discovery of long-acting sulphamides may permit the reduction of medical intervention to a single injection" (Lapeyssonnie, Momenteau, 1961; Lapeyssonnie, Chabbert, Bonnardot, et al., 1961; Lapeyssonnie, Bonnardot, Louis, et al., 1961). In practice, it was indeed difficult to give oral antibiotics three times a day to thousands of patients, some of them in comas, and spread over potentially large distances. This is why the development of a long-acting intramuscular sulphamide, Sultirene, was a significant step forward in treatment—due to its efficacy and ease of use (Chippaux, 2001).

Sadly, the use of this drug was quickly compromised. Fewer than ten years after its development, the first resistances appeared. By the beginning of the 1970s the sulphamides were no longer sufficiently efficacious, and classical seven- to ten-day treatments were difficult to administer in practice.

Michel Rey, back in France after a long spell in West Africa, where he had been in charge of the Infectious Diseases department at Dakar Hospital, became involved in the research and development of short treatments for meningococcal meningitis. Inspired by Yves Chabbert at the Pasteur Institute (who collaborated with Lapeyssonnie on long-acting sulphamides) and Jacques Acar, Rey launched a new single-dose treatment—oily chloramphenicol by intramuscular injection. Once the dosage form was perfected, Rey and his team tested the treatment in several West African countries. Encouraging initial results were obtained in Dakar and Ouagadougou (Rey et al., 1975). The study was completed by looking at 74 consecutive meningitis cases in Bobo-Dioulasso, treated by single injection of oily chloramphenicol. The results obtained in 1976 led the authors to propose chloramphenicol in oily suspension as an alternative to long-acting sulphamides in epidemics of cerebrospinal meningitis epidemics, and also as initial treatment for endemic and sporadic cases in rural African settings (Rey et al., 1976).

The efficacy of oral and intravenous chloramphenicol in the treatment of meningococcal meningitis had already been studied (Girgis et al., 1972; Whittle et al., 1973). The development of a long-acting intramuscular injection dosage form, however, allowed single-dose treatments. Following the results of this study, oily chloramphenicol was registered in France and produced by Roussel Laboratories.

Epicentre's Contribution to the Prescription of Oily Chloramphenicol and Ceftriaxone in Africa

The first major epidemic outbreak occurred in countries that are part of the so-called "meningitis belt" between 1987 and 1989. Sudan was particularly affected in 1988, followed by Ethiopia in 1989, reporting thirty-two thousand and forty-one thousand cases respectively (WHO, 1998). MSF opened a mission in Sudan in 1988 and proposed oily chloramphenicol for curative care of meningitis cases. The treatment protocol was refused by Sudanese authorities as it did not correspond to national guidelines. MSF teams were thus forced to use ampicillin injections over several days. A doctor from the mission explained that "half the patients left before finishing treatment. It was just impossible. The teams were going out of their minds."

Medical practice and research in English-speaking countries evolved more quickly towards evidence-based medicine than in French-speaking countries. Treatments and therapeutic protocols were studied according to international biomedical criteria and communicated through publication in reputed medical journals.

The single-dose oily chloramphenicol protocol was unheard of in the former British colonies at the time, despite being in everyday use in French-speaking countries. Clinical trials carried out on the molecule did not provide sufficient proof as far as criteria in English-speaking countries were concerned. As far as we know, only four studies can be found in medical literature before 1988, two of which were performed by Rey's team in Saliou, in Senegal, and Ouedraogo, in Burkina Faso (1975, 1976), and published in French journals. The other two were written by one English-speaking group (Wali et al., 1979; Puddicombe, Wali, Greenwood, 1984). Results were comparable: (1) oily chloramphenicol seemed just as efficacious as longer, classical treatments; (2) the single- or two-injection protocols were significantly advantageous in resource-limited countries; (3) the low cost of treatment also made it more affordable in these countries; (4) theoretical chloramphenicol toxicity appears negligible when compared with the morbidity and mortality of meningococcal disease, particularly during epidemics. In short, this protocol appeared to be a promising first-line treatment option in developing countries. None of these studies provided "scientific approval" according to the standards in English-speaking countries, however. In all four studies, the numbers of patients studied were too low to provide statistically significant results, and only two were published in English.

MSF senior staff members were quickly convinced of the need for progress. They knew from their own experience that chloramphenicol was easier to use and efficacious. According to field doctors, this drug needed to be available for use in all meningococcal meningitis epidemics, including in East Africa. The experience in Sudan demonstrated the need to perform an efficacy study according to international scientific norms.

The study protocol, written by an Epicentre epidemiologist, was applied in two referral hospitals in Niamey and Bamako, in collaboration with Nigerien and Malian health authorities. An unblinded, random controlled trial of 515 patients compared the clinical and biological efficacy of two injections of oily chlor-amphenicol with the previous standard, which involved eight days of intravenous ampicillin.

Results showed comparable efficacy for the two treatments. Given feasibility and cost criteria, the authors recommended the use of oily chloramphenicol as first-line treatment for bacterial meningitides in peripheral health structures in the Sudan–Sahel region. They also added that better chloramphenicol pharma-cokinetics studies were required to optimize treatment efficacy, and, furthermore, that high mortality rates should motivate further research for new, better, simple-to-use treatments such as ceftriaxone (Varaine, 1990).

The study was published in *The Lancet* in 1991 (Pécoul, Varaine, Keita, et al., 1991). These results scientifically validated the protocol and led to its worldwide transmission. Oily chloramphenicol use quickly became widespread in former British colonies following the publication of this article (it was used in 1991 in Uganda, for example), and became the rule, as shown by national protocols in the Sudan–Sahel region from this time on.

In terms of international health policy, the World Health Organization (WHO) put oily chloramphenicol on its essential drugs list, then subsequently recommended it in its first guide on controlling meningitis epidemics (WHO, 1995). It became the recommended first-line treatment a few years later, in 1997, after the creation of the International Coordinating Group on Vaccine Provision for Epidemic Meningitis Control (ICG), and still is today.

The drug is not fully accepted by some scientists and officials, however. Its toxicity in oral and intravenous use has been criticized, and the drug was pulled from the European market after a number of cases of bone marrow aplasia in richer countries. This led the original manufacturer, Roussel, to halt production. The International Dispensary Association (IDA) started production after calls from MSF, but transferred production to an Indian pharmacological laboratory following technical production difficulties. This company is still the only oily chloramphenicol manufacturer in the world.

Some countries in the meningitis belt have categorically refused to use the drug, despite WHO recommendations, because it was seen as "a drug for poor countries." There is often confusion with respect to the benefits of this particular dosage form and the use of the molecule in general. Over and above occasional refusals to use the drug, lack of knowledge also leads to doubts about its inclusion on the WHO essential drugs list.

Finally, an alternative exists: the third-generation cephalosporin ceftriaxone. During the 1990s, this drug was too expensive for use in resource-limited countries, particularly in such large-scale public health interventions as meningitis epidemics.

MSF's involvement in ceftriaxone use began early, through a randomized double-blind trial in 1991 comparing the efficacy of two injections of either oily chloramphenicol or ceftriaxone in the treatment of bacterial meningitis. The study was carried out in Niamey and Bamako between 1991 and 1995, and the study population included children of two to thirty-five months of age, suffering from purulent bacterial meningitis (all germs). The results suggested that two injections of ceftriaxone were more efficacious in reducing mortality than two doses of oily chloramphenicol. The study authors publicly requested the immediate availability of cheaper generic ceftriaxone for use in resource-limited countries (Varaine et al., 1997). This position was restated at international conferences and expert working groups, such as the Eighth Infectious Diseases Conference in Boston in 1998 (Varaine, Keita, Kaninda, et al., 1998).

The significance of the study results was somewhat limited, however. The study did not question the use of oily chloramphenicol, nor did it examine efficacy during epidemics. The study was not carried out during epidemic periods, and only a third of cases were meningococcal.

In 2002, facing increasing difficulties in the supply of oily chloramphenicol, and with the price of ceftriaxone progressive reduced, MSF and Epicentre decided to proceed with an equivalence study comparing oily chloramphenicol and ceftriaxone.

The way this study was set up in the field is a good example of MSF's specific potential. The aim was to recruit enough patients during an epidemic,[1] which, according to a senior Epicentre staff member, involved "being in the right place at the right time." The four selected countries for the study were Chad, Mali, Niger, and Burkina Faso. Preliminary negotiations to obtain agreements from the health authorities were successful except in Burkina Faso. An epidemic then began in Burkina Faso at the start of winter 2003. The MSF and Epicentre team immediately left for the site, but authorizations were slow to arrive. Senior MSF staff in Paris then asked their team to go to neighboring Niger. A few days later, the epidemic hit the Zinder region and spread to Maradi, where the research team was in place and waiting, supported by regular regional MSF field teams; the study could be started, and 510 meningitis patients were subsequently recruited for the cohort. The results showed no inferiority of ceftriaxone when compared with oily chloramphenicol when both are used as short treatments for meningococcal meningitis. The authors conclude that ceftriaxone is an equivalent alternative to chloramphenicol for epidemic responses (Nathan et al., 2005). The specificity of this study was that it was conducted during an *epidemic*.

The study required a significant amount of technical input from MSF. MSF's logistics potential was a major asset, and the presence of MSF teams across the region and locally, in this case in Maradi, provided material and technical support for research teams. Logistical coordination was another key factor during this intervention, both in material and medical logistics (particularly laboratory services in the case of meningitis epidemics). Furthermore, the absence of institutional administrative and diplomatic red tape allowed for reactivity and flexibility that are not to be found in most state or United Nations bodies. Nor

---

1   Reminder: meningitis belt epidemics only last from a few weeks to a couple of months, and over five hundred patients needed to be recruited for the study.

did this autonomy undermine interactions with collaborating partners: effective and efficacious collaboration was built with national institutions, particularly the Medical and Sanitary Research Centre of Niger and Nigerien health authorities.

In 2008, both treatment protocols validated by MSF became international standards for meningococcal meningitis outbreaks in the meningitis belt region. The availability of these two drugs means that sporadic cases and epidemic outbreaks can be treated. Both are of significant clinical benefit in the treatment of meningococcal meningitis.

Vaccines and Vaccination Strategies

The first trials of anti-meningococcal vaccines were held in Sudan in 1915, but all efforts to put them into use were in vain until the 1960s. Gotschlich, Goldschneider, and Artenstein, working for a United States Army research institute, were the first to extract and purify the A and C polysaccharides. Their work demonstrated the immunogenicity of these polysaccharides in man (Gotschlich et al., 1969). A monovalent C polysaccharide vaccine was quickly developed for the United States, where this serogroup predominates. The first trials were performed in 1970 in US Army training centers, where regular outbreaks occurred (Artenstein et al., 1970).

This new technology quickly crossed the Atlantic to French-speaking Africa. In 1970–71, Emil Gotschlich and Charles Mérieux collaborated to produce a vaccine providing protection against the meningococcal serogroup A, directly followed by a study of immune response in cohorts of adults in the United States and children in Dakar (Emil Gotschlich and Michel Rey). The study demonstrated serogroup A vaccine immunogenicity, although the results suggested that this was lesser than that of the C serogroup vaccine. The study also reported that immu-

114

nogenicity was very poor in infants aged six to thirteen months (Gotschlich, Rey, Triau, Sparks, 1972; Gotschlich, Rey, Etienne, et al., 1972).

The Mérieux Institute launched vaccine production. Lapeyssonnie, working for the WHO in Alexandria, supported the first controlled trials performed in Egypt in 1972 (Wadhan et al., 1973) and in Sudan in 1973 (Erwa et al., 1973). Immediately following these studies, Charles Mérieux and Lapeyssonnie entrusted the vaccine to Pierre Saliou's team at the Biology Department of the Muraz Centre in Bobo-Dioulasso. During the outbreaks in Mali and Upper Volta in 1974, Saliou and his team put into place vaccination campaigns to compensate for sulfamide resistance in African strains of Neisseria *meningitidis*. The campaigns were deemed a success (Saliou, Stoeckel, Lafaye, et al., 1978).

Description of Initial Vaccination Strategies

Epidemic control measures were transformed by the arrival of these new anti-meningococcal vaccines (monovalent A and C and bivalent AC). Lapeyssonnie immediately proposed a guide to their use at the International Seminar on Immunization, in Bamako, 1974 (Lapeyssonnie, 1970; Lapeyssonnie, 1974). Pierre Saliou and Philippe Stoeckel's team then performed several studies defining the main elements of a "circumstantial" vaccination strategy (Saliou et al., 1978; Saliou, Rey, Stoeckel, 1978; Yada et al., 1983).

This strategy is based on epidemiological surveillance at peripheral health centers during the epidemic season. As soon as the first cases are reported, two interventions occur: curative care (treatment of sick patients) to reduce mortality; and the identification of the serogroup involved; with an ensuing circumstantial vaccination campaign targeting the affected population to stop the spread of the epidemic.

Circumstantial vaccination is a reactive approach. Given that the polysaccharide vaccine is only immunogenic from two years of age, its inclusion as a blanket protective measure in expanded programs of immunization was not feasible. A reactive strategy targets children aged eighteen months through to adults aged thirty years in the affected region, starting as quickly as possible once the first cases are confirmed[2]. The most affected area is the first priority, and vaccination coverage progressively extends to neighboring areas in expanding concentric circles. The problem is being sensitive enough to react as quickly as possible, but specific enough not to launch unnecessary campaigns because the human and financial inputs for mass vaccination are often to the detriment of curative care. In other words, the main difficulty resides in the sensitivity and specificity in detection thresholds used.

Several years passed before the first reference study regarding detection thresholds was performed, however. A Centers for Disease Control and Prevention (CDC)[3] team at the beginning of the 1990s analyzed data gathered between 1979 and 1984 in the Burkina Faso epidemiological surveillance system. Because vaccination response depends on the rapidity and the reliability of epidemic detection, the authors proposed an evaluation of the usefulness of a weekly incidence rate using retrospective analysis. The results suggest acceptable sensitivity and specificity for a threshold of fifteen cases per one hundred thousand inhabitants per week averaged over two weeks for populations of at least thirty thousand to fifty thousand, and of five cases per one hundred thousand inhabitants per week for zones neighboring epidemic outbreaks. According to the authors, given the rudimentary nature of data collected in Sahel countries'

2 Initial studies having shown poor group A vaccine immunogenicity in infants, early recommendations proposed excluding them from vaccination campaigns.

3 The CDC, based in Atlanta, in the USA, is one of the thirteen main US Department of Health and Human Services agencies.

surveillance systems, these measures were acceptable to detect epidemic emergencies. They underlined, however, that further studies were required to examine the appropriateness of these recommended thresholds (Moore et al., 1992).

The CDC team's conclusions quickly became an international standard. In its first *Practical Guidelines for Control of Epidemic Meningococcal Disease*, the WHO cited the study results, which subsequently became official recommendations in epidemic detection and for launching mass vaccination campaigns (WHO, 1995).

Several retrospective analyses of epidemic responses have progressively called into question the thresholds defined by the CDC team, however. Furthermore, worldwide anti-meningococcal vaccine shortages during the 1996 outbreak in Nigeria were decisive in changing the face of vaccination strategies.

MSF Meningitis Vaccination Experience

MSF intervened regularly in meningitis belt countries during the 1980s, where teams were confronted by meningitis epidemics. The organization employed the strategies established by the pioneers of meningitis vaccination in Africa the preceding decade. Circumstantial vaccination campaigns spreading concentrically from outbreak zones were the rule, such as during the Ugandan epidemic in 1982-83.

At the same time, MSF missions were progressively supported by the headquarters' medical department and Epicentre. The first field experiences, considered in the light of improving technical analysis, along with capacity-building from centrally documented experiences, led to questions about internationally accepted practices.

MSF missions involving responses to meningitis epidemics multiplied during the 1990s, mostly in direct collaboration with national health authorities. Nineteen missions between 1990 and 1999 were formally analyzed by MSF and Epicentre, and these descriptive studies supplied quantitative data about the epidemiology of the disease, as well as the effect of responses put in place by national health authorities and NGOs. In 1993 the first two guidelines were published (Epicentre, Varaine, 1993a,b).

The results of these analyses often suggest a weak effect, if any at all, of vaccination campaigns on overall epidemic progression. For MSF meningitis specialists, it became increasingly apparent that preventive measures to control the disease needed reviewing. Initially, vaccination strategies dating from the 1970s were re-adapted. The "concentric circle" strategy was gradually abandoned in favor of urban agglomeration outbreak vaccination. These kinds of strategies were based on careful compromises between curative and preventive interventions. Simply put, curative care was decentralized with adequate peripheral drug stocks, and vaccination efforts were concentrated on the largest demographic areas hit by the epidemic. Later, for example in 1996, during the outbreaks in which Nigeria was hardest hit, the need to adapt vaccination strategies became apparent.

Meningitis cases began to be reported in North and East Nigeria in December 1995. By the beginning of February, increasing disease incidence was reported to the national health authorities. The Ministry of Health reinforced the vaccination campaign that had already been launched, and organized an evaluation in affected districts. On February 13, 1996, an MSF team arrived in the country for an exploratory mission to work alongside the government team and the accompanying WHO and United Nations Children's Fund (UNICEF) staff to evaluate the outbreak in the northern and central regions of Nigeria. The mission confirmed a meningitis epidemic outbreak and identified *N. meningitidis* serogroup A as the causal agent. In four states, 7,400 cases and 1,560 deaths were reported in the first two months of 1996, a specific mortality rate of 20%. MSF decided to establish a mission to support government vaccination activities, curative care, and surveillance-system reinforcement in the three most affected states—a population of fourteen million. The emergency mission grew rapidly and involved the recruitment of several dozen international staff, the participation of all five MSF operational centers, and the emergency supply of several tons of medical equipment. From March to May almost three million people were vaccinated and more than thirty thousand cases treated. A worldwide shortage of vaccine stocks followed.

As the epidemic developed, MSF requested an external evaluation of the intervention by the European Agency for Development and Health (AEDES).[4] Their conclusions raised the same questions MSF specialists had been asking previously. Prevention strategies put into action were compromised by a surveillance system that provided inadequate data in terms of rapidity and reliability: the mass vaccination campaign's effect was probably weak because it was introduced too late. Although the authors underlined the fact that the results were impressive in terms of the number of people vaccinated and treated, it still appeared painfully obvious that the results obtained were not equal to the significant means employed to achieve them (Farese et al., 1996).

International Health Politics, a New Type of Collaboration Between MSF and the WHO

For the majority of meningitis specialists, including those at the WHO and MSF, the 1996 crisis showed the need to organize a coordinated international response to better confront future epidemics. At the time, WHO reports were asking the same questions about vaccination strategies as those elucidated in MSF–Epicentre studies. The WHO brought together the world's

---

4   The AEDES is "a consulting firm, specialized in the Food, Social and Public Health sector," and a regular Epicentre collaborator.

major players in meningitis in Geneva, December 1996. Participants included the CDC, UNICEF, the International Cooperation Agency for Preventive Medicine (AMP),[5] the International Federation of Red Cross and Red Crescent Societies (IFRC), MSF, and various scientific specialists. A funding appeal signed by the WHO, UNICEF, the IFRC, and MSF was subsequently launched. The ICG was created in January 1997. Additional technical partners were added to the core organization (the CDC, the Tropical Medicine Institute of the Military Health Service in Marseille,, and the National Public Health Institute in Oslo), as well as vaccine manufacturers.

The first objective of the newly created ICG was to evaluate vaccine needs in meningitis belt countries and compare these with available international resources. Group members immediately entered into discussions with vaccine manufacturers to guarantee minimum stock levels and costs for epidemic responses. After estimating epidemic season needs for 1997, a joint international appeal was launched in February for the $6.4 million needed by ICG members. The funds obtained paid for stocks of the first bivalent A C combined vaccines reserves produced by the two manufacturers at the time: GlaxoSmithKline (GSK) and Pasteur-Mérieux (later Aventis-Pasteur, then Sanofi Pasteur). Authorization procedures were created to regulate stock distributions. When receiving a request from a Sahel-region country, the four members of the ICG guaranteed a consultative answer within forty-eight hours, and supply depending on epidemic risk criteria and proposed vaccination strategies. The key issues for ICG members were to evaluate vaccination campaign appropriateness and to guarantee rational use of supplied vaccines. In 1997–98, over half of the vaccines supplied to Africa were sourced from the ICG (WHO, 1997).

---

5   The AMP is a non-governmental association created by Charles Mérieux and Jacques Monod in 1972. It aims to constitute a relay between research progress and its application in the field.

Over and above vaccines and injection material, the ICG also secured stocks of oily chloramphenicol as production was regularly threatened. To complete the list of tools required for epidemic response, the ICG proposed diagnostic and epidemiological follow-up material (latex agglutination tests, transport, and culture media). Furthermore, the group recruited new partners, creating a worldwide meningitis network, the "greater ICG" that meets once a year. Discussion topics include the evaluation of epidemic responses over the preceding year, technical and scientific progress, and future response planning.

Redefining Detection Thresholds

Analyses of the interventions in African countries in the 1990s suggested that epidemic detection was inadequate for effective preventive control. MSF tries to systematically evaluate its interventions, and each time the evaluation authors question the effect of vaccination campaigns, as seen in the numerous reports by Epicentre and several articles published in the international medical press (Barrand et al., 1993; Lewis et al., 2001). External audits reach the same conclusions: the efficacy of preventive measures with respect to epidemic curve progress is questioned and the cost-benefit ratio often appears unfavorable (Lengeler et al., 1995; Woods et al., 2000; Veeken et al., 1998). As a key actor supporting countries in mass vaccination campaigns, MSF missions in this domain are regularly criticized.

In 1999 the ICG mandated MSF to report on the progress of field research into epidemic thresholds for meningitis. In June 2000 MSF and Epicentre met in Paris with international research teams and public health actors from affected countries to draft new recommendations for meningitis epidemic detection in Africa. The experts present agreed that the threshold of fifteen cases per one hundred thousand inhabitants a week averaged over two weeks was very specific in confirming a meningitis epidemic. They nevertheless explained that this indicator has several limits: (1) it is not sufficiently sensitive to detect all epidemics; (2) the delay between crossing the threshold value and the epidemic peak is too short (less than three weeks) to perform a mass vaccination campaign; (3) under-reporting and case-declaration delays in affected countries' surveillance systems reduced threshold sensitivity and significantly contributed to delays in the detection of epidemics. The need to use lower epidemic threshold values to allow sufficient time for mass vaccination campaigns was recognized. To avoid false alerts, however, the recommendations are adjusted according to the context in which they are applied. Contextual elements to be taken into account include recent or ongoing meningitis epidemics in the region, calculated meningitis vaccination coverage, the time of year, population size and density, and surveillance system quality.

These new recommendations define an alert threshold to launch investigations and begin preparations for a meningitis epidemic, and an epidemic threshold, confirming an epidemic and reinforcing control measures. For each threshold, a series of actions are suggested according to epidemic risk and population size and density. Where there have been no recent epidemics, or in areas where vaccination coverage is low, the lowest threshold is recommended. In an epidemic context, attaining alert levels is sufficient to launch a full epidemic response. These new recommendations provide a general framework for meningitis epidemic detection and responses in highly endemic African countries (Epicentre, 2000).

The WHO validated this meeting's recommendations and embraced them as official policy. It then transmitted the new recommendations through international ICG meetings and WHO publications (WHO, 2000).

For MSF meningitis specialists, the June 2000 meeting led to changes in how detection thresholds are perceived. A new notion was born: the idea of geographical control of epidemic spread. If the first outbreak is difficult to recognize in time, adjusted thresholds can serve as quality indicators of epidemic spread to adjacent areas. When actors are alerted of an outbreak, surveillance is reinforced and detection thresholds can then reach acceptable sensitivity. For MSF specialists, this new approach promised to lead to better control of meningitis epidemics in Africa (Lewis, Nathan, Communier, et al., 2001).

The Emergence of the N. Meningitidis W135 Serogroup

A new wave of epidemics occurred in 2001, particularly in Burkina Faso and Niger, and the Pasteur Institute and AMP began a joint exploratory mission. The results showed the highest levels of the W135 serogroup ever recorded in Africa (Taha et al., 2002; Châtelet et al., 2002). The dominant A serogroup vied for the first time in meningitis belt countries with the W135 strain, found in 38% of investigated cases in Burkina Faso and 39% in Niger.

The survey's conclusions immediately raised new questions about the evolving epidemiological landscape and vaccination strategies, even if it was clear that the A serogroup continued to dominate other countries in the region. Before the appearance of W135, vaccination campaigns used bivalent AC vaccines, with stocks guaranteed by the ICG. At that time, only two vaccine manufacturers produced tetravalent ACYW135 polysaccharide vaccine effective against the W135 strain. Given the high cost of this vaccine and limited production capacity, its large-scale public health use in Africa was not feasible. MSF reacted quickly to the new situation, and senior staff members established initially informal contacts with one of the pharmaceutical companies producing the tetravalent vaccine, GSK. Following these initial discussions, expert meetings were organized involving ICG members and GSK representatives. Two possibilities are discussed: a monovalent W135 vaccine, or a trivalent ACW135 product. The second option was chosen, and GSK agreed to start production on the condition of prepayment for a minimum of six million doses. MSF contributed €2 million, and enlisted other ICG partners. GSK began production, and Belgian government authorities, under pressure from all partners, registered the product in record time. Continuing the same frenetic pace, the WHO, GSK, and the CDC performed a trial in Burkina Faso to validate large-scale use of the product. A few months after the first W135 epidemic in 2001, the new vaccine was available for use in meningitis belt countries and quickly employed. The following year, a new W135 epidemic hit Burkina Faso, and the WHO reported the first large-scale epidemic due to the strain since its arrival in Africa the previous year (Bertherat et al., 2002).

Since 2002, no major W135 epidemic has occurred, and the ICG still has more than half of its initial vaccine stocks (around 2.5 million were used out of the 6 million doses delivered). The epidemiological history of potential strains (including W135) does suggest, however, that new large-scale epidemics may soon occur (Traoré et al., 2006). Strain variations underline the importance of regular serogroup surveillance by field actors sending samples to reference laboratories in Oslo and Marseille.

The WHO and MSF have transformed meningitis control policy through the mediation of the ICG, an innovative public health–intervention action group of a type that has since gained widespread acceptance. It has been a model for yellow fever control (the Yellow Fever ICG) and for the fight against drug-resistant tuberculosis (the Green Light Committee).

The sequence of practices developed by MSF in meningitis epidemic responses is one example amongst others of the specific nature of the institution's evolution. With the exception of the first chloramphenicol trial in 1989, MSF intervened throughout the 1980s and 1990s first and foremost as a field practitioner. MSF's efforts were focused on curative care for affected populations in collaboration with local health authorities. Solid scientific evidence was produced based on field experience, which MSF used in another sphere of action, that of international health policy. The WHO and MSF worked together, in a new kind of collaboration, and defined new meningitis control strategies. As such, MSF became a recommender of new international health policy alongside the WHO.

Bibliography

Artenstein, M. S., R. Gold, J.G Zimmerly, F.A. Wyle, H. Schneider, C. Harkins. 1970. "Prevention of meningococcal disease by group C polysaccharide vaccine." *The New England Journal of Medicine* 282: 417–420.

Barret, B., T. Ancelle, L. Flachet, I. Harndt, J. Castilla, A. Moren. 1993. "Epidémie de méningite à méningocoque à Moyo, Ouganda, 1991–1992: investigation et stratégie d'intervention." *Cahiers Santé* 3 (2): 98–103.

Bertherat, E., A. Yada, M. H. Djinbarey, B. Koumare. 2002. "Première épidémie de grande ampleur provoquée par *Neisseria meningitidis* W135 en Afrique." *Médecine tropicale* 62 (3): 301–304.

Châtelet, I. P., J. M. Alonso, M. K. Tah. 2002. "Clonal expansion of *Neisseria meningitidis* W135. Epidemiological implications for the African meningitis belt." *Bulletin de la Société de Pathologie Exotique* 95 (5): 323–324.

Chippaux, A. 2001. "Lapeyssonnie nous a quittés." *Bulletin de la Société de Pathologie Exotique* 94 (4): 291–292.

Epicentre, F. Varaine. 1993a. *Épidémie de méningite. Guide pratique pour les agents de santé.* Epicentre.

Epicentre, F. Varaine. 1993b. *Conduite à tenir en cas d'épidémie de méningite. Manuel pratique à l'usage des DPS et DCS.* Epicentre.

Epicentre. 2000. *Réunion de consensus sur la détection des épidémies de méningite en Afrique, 20 juin 2000.* Unpublished report. Epicentre.

Erwa, H. H., M.A. Haseeb, A.A. Idris, L. Lapeyssonnie, W.R. Sanborn, J.E. Sippel. 1973. "A serogroup A meningococcal poly-saccharide vaccine: studies in the Sudan to combat cerebro-spinal meningitis caused by Neisseria meningitidis group A." *Bulletin of the World Health Organization* 49: 301–305.

Farese, P., A. Procuret Blaustein, J. Margets. 1996. *Meningitis epidemic in Nigeria, 1996. Evaluation of the MSF operation in North Nigeria from February to May 1996.* Unpublished report. European Agency for Development and Health.

Girgis, N. I., M.W. Yassin, W.R. Sanborn, R.E. Burdick, H.A. el-Ela, D.C. Kent, K. Sorenson, I.M. Nabil. 1972. "Ampicillin compared with penicillin and chloramphenicol combined in the treatment of bacterial meningitis." *Journal of Tropical Medicine & Hygiene* 75 (8): 154–157.

Gotschlich, E. C., I. Goldschneider, M. S. Artenstein. 1969. "Human immunity to the meningococcus IV. Immunogenicity of group A and group C polysaccharides in human volunteers." *The Journal of Experimental Medicine.* 129: 1367–1384.

Gotschlich, E. C., M. Rey, R. Triau, K. J. Sparks. 1972. "Quantitative determination of the human immune response to immunization with Meningococcal Vaccines." *The Journal of Clinical Investigation* 51 (1): 89–96.

Gotschlich, E. C., M. Rey, J. Etienne, W.R. Sanborn, R. Triau, B. Cvjetanovic. 1972. "The immunological responses observed in field studies in Africa with group A meningococcal vaccines." *Progress in Immunobiological Standardization* 5: 485–491.

Lapeyssonnie, L., H. Momenteau. 1961. "Note sur 19 souches de Neisseria intracellularis isolées au Niger en 1961." *Médecine tropicale* 21: 526–530.

Lapeyssonnie, L., Y. Chabbert, R. Bonnardot, M. Lefevre, J. Louis. 1961. "Clinical and biological data concerning the treatment of cerebrospinal meningitis by sulfamethoxypyridazine. Results observed after a single intramuscular injection." *Bulletin de la Société de Pathologie Exotique* 54: 955–976.

Lapeyssonnie, L., R. Bonnardot, J. Louis, M. Lefevre. 1961. "First note concerning the activity of a single dose of sulfamethoxypyrinamide by intramuscular route in the treatment of meningococcal cerebrospinal meningitis." *Médecine tropicale* 21: 129–133.

Lapeyssonnie, L. 1970. "De quelques problèmes pratiques posés par les essais contrôlés sur le terrain d'un vaccin anti-méningococcoque." *Médecine tropicale*. 30: 624–628.

——. 1974. "Stratégie d'emploi des vaccins antiméningococciques." *Séminaire international sur les vaccinations en Afrique, Bamako, novembre 1974*, 183–189. Éditions Fondation Mérieux.

Lengeler, C., W. Kessler, D. Daugla. 1995. "The 1990 meningococcal meningitis epidemic of Sarh: how useful was an earlier mass vaccination?" *Acta Tropica* 59 (3): 211–222.

Lewis, R., N. Nathan, L. Diarra, F. Belanger, C. Paquet. 2001. "Timely detection of meningococcal meningitis epidemics in Africa." *The Lancet* 358 (9278): 287–293.

Lewis, R., N. Nathan, A. Communier, F. Varaine, F. Fermon, F. De Chabalier, N. Rosenstein, M. Djingarey, L. Diarra, A. Yada, E. Tikhomirov, M. Santamaria, M. Hardiman, D. Legros. 2001. "Mieux détecter les épidémies de méningite à méningocoque en Afrique: une nouvelle recommandation." *Cahiers Santé* 11 (4): 251–255.

Moore, P. S., B. D. Plikaytis, G. A. Bolan, M.J. Oxtoby, A. Yada, A. Zoubga, A.L. Reingold, C.V. Broome. 1992. "Detection of meningitis epidemics in Africa: a population-based analysis." *International Journal of Epidemiology* 21 (1): 155–162.

Nathan, N., T. Borel, A. Djibo, D. Evans, S. Djibo, J.F. Corty, M. Guillerm, K.P. Alberti, L. Pinoges, P.J. Guerin, D. Legros. 2005. "Ceftriaxone as effective as long-acting chloramphenicol in short-course treatment of meningococcal meningitis during epidemics: a randomised non-inferiority study." *The Lancet* 366 (9482): 308–313.

Pécoul, B., F. Varaine, M. Keita, G. Soga, A. Djibo, G. Soula, A. Abdou, J. Etienne, M. Rey. 1991. "Long-acting chloramphenicol versus intravenous ampicillin for treatment of bacterial meningitis." *The Lancet* 338: 862–866.

Puddicombe, J. B., S. S. Wali, B. M. Greenwood. 1984. "A field trial of a single intramuscular injection of long-acting chloramphenicol in the treatment of meningococcal meningitis." *Transactions of the Royal Society of Tropical Medicine and Hygiene* 78 (3): 399–409.

Rey, M., J. Acar, I. Diop-Mar et al. 1975. "Lettre: méningite méningococcique cérébro-spinale en Afrique. Traitement par injection unique intra-musculaire de chloramphénicol (suspension huileuse)." *Nouvelle Presse Médicale* 4 (17): 1289.

Rey, M., L. Ouegraogo, P. Saliou, L. Perino. 1976. "Traitement minute de la méningite cérébro-spinale épidémique par injection intra-musculaire unique de chloramphénicol (suspension huileuse)." *Médecine et Maladies infectieuses* 6 (4): 120–124.

Saliou, P., Ph. Stoeckel, A. Lafaye, J.L Rey, J. Renaudet. 1978. "Essais contrôlés du vaccin antiméningococcique polysaccharidique A en Afrique de l'Ouest Sahélienne (Haute-Volta et Mali)." *Developments in Biological Standardization* 41: 97–108.

Saliou P., J.-L. Rey, Ph. Stoeckel. 1978. "Une nouvelle stratégie de lutte contre les épidémies de méningite à méningocoque en

Afrique sahélienne." *Bulletin de la Société de Pathologie Exotique* 71: 34–45.

Taha, M.-K., I. Parent du Chatelet, M. Schlumberger, I Sanou, S. Djibo, F. De Chabalier, J-M Alonso. 2002. "Neisseria meningitidis serogroup W135 and A were equally prevalent among meningitis cases occurring at the end of the 2001 epidemics in Burkina Faso and Niger." *Journal of Clinical Microbiology* 40 (3): 1083–1084.

Traoré, Y., B.-M. Njanpop-Lafourcade, K.-L.-S. Adjogble, M. Lourde, S. Yaro, B. Nacro, A. Drabo, I. Parent du Chatelet, J.E. Mueller, M-K Taha, R. Borrow, P. Nicolas, J-M Alonso, B.D. Gessner. 2006. "The rise and fall of epidemic Neisseria meningitidis serogroup W135 meningitis in Burkina Faso, 2002–2005." *Clinical Infectious Diseases* 43 (7): 817–822.

Varaine, F. 1990. *Essai clinique comparant une double injection de chloramphénicol huileux à l'ampicilline dans le traitement des méningites bactériennes.* Unpublished report. Epicentre.

Varaine, F., A. V. Kaninda, B. Pécoul, C. Paquet, A. Moren. 1997. *Essai clinique comparant la ceftriaxone et le chloramphénicol huileux dans le traitement des méningites bactériennes chez les enfants de 2 à 35 mois au Mali et au Niger.* Unpublished report. Epicentre

Varaine, F., M. Keita, A. V. Kaninda, et al. 1998. "Long acting chloramphenicol versus ceftriaxone for treatment of bacterial meningitis in children aged 2–35 months." Eighth International Congress for Infectious Diseases, Boston, Maryland, May 15–18, 1998.

Veeken, H., K. Ritmeijer, B. Hausman. 1998. "Priority during a meningitis epidemic: vaccination or treatment." *Bulletin of the World Health Organization* 76 (2): 135–141.

Wali, S. S., J. T. MacFarlane, W. R. Weir. 1979. "Single injection treatment of meningococcal meningitis. 2. Long-acting chloramphenicol." *Transactions of the Royal Society of Tropical Medicine and Hygiene* 73 (6): 698–702.

Wadhan, M. H., S.A. Sallam, M.N. Hassan, A. Abdel Gawad, A.S Rakha, J.E Sippel, R. Hablas, W.R. Sanborn, N.M Kassem, S.M. Riad, B Cvjetanovic. 1973. "A controlled field trial of a serogroup A meningococcal polysaccharide vaccine." *Bulletin of the World Health Organization* 48: 667–673.

Whittle, H. C., N.M. Davidson, B.M Greenwood, D.A.Warrell, A. Tomkins, P. Tugwell, A. Zalin, A.D Bryceson, E.H Parry, M. Brueton, M. Duggan, A.D. Rajkovic. 1973. "Trial of chloramphenicol for meningitis in northern savanna of Africa." *British Medical Journal* 3 (5876): 379–81.

World Health Organization (WHO). 1995, *Control of epidemic meningococcal disease. WHO practical guidelines.* Dardilly: Fondation Marcel Mérieux.

——. 1997. "Response to epidemic meningitis in Africa, 1997." *Weekly Epidemiological Record*, 72 (42): 313–318.

——. 1998. *Control of epidemic meningococcal disease. WHO practical guidelines*, 2nd edition, Genève: World Health Organization.

——. 2000. "Détecter une épidémie de méningite à méningocoque dans les pays à forte endémicité en Afrique. Recommandation de l'OMS." *Relevé épidémiogique hebdomadaire* 75 (38): 306–309.

Woods, C. W., G. Armstrong, S. Sackey, C. Tetteh, S. Bugri, B.A. Perkins, N.E Rosenstein. 2000. "Emergency vaccination against epidemic meningitis in Ghana: implication for the control of meningococcal disease in West Africa." *The Lancet* 355 (9197): 30–33.

Yada, A. A., P. Saliou, P. Stoeckel, J. Roux. 1983. "La vaccination de circonstance préventive, variant dans la stratégie de lutte contre la méningite cérébro-spinale à méningocoque." *Médecine tropicale* 43: 219–222.

Chapter 7

Human African Trypanosomiasis

Stopping the Use of Arsenic

Jean-François Corty

Human African trypanosomiasis (more commonly known as sleeping sickness) was a frequent scourge of the colonial period, but virtually disappeared in the years following independence. It made a comeback in the closing decades of the twentieth century, however, and now affects between 50,000 and 150,000 people a year, and threatens nearly 50 million. Thanks to improved surveillance since the early 1990s, the post-colonial epidemic now appears under control. Where before there were high-prevalence foci, there are now numerous minor foci scattered throughout Africa's tsetse fly belt.

Aside from its unique pathophysiology, what makes this disease so serious is the insidious and potentially devastating dynamic of outbreaks (Cattand, 2001, p. 315). These occur primarily in the Democratic Republic of Congo (DRC), Angola, and southern Sudan, although the Congo Republic, Ivory Coast, Tanzania, and the Central African Republic also report some cases. With no existing vaccine and a prevalence that can exceed 50% in places, it's not rare for trypanosomiasis to be the most common, or second most common, cause of death in certain communities, ahead of HIV/AIDS (Courtin, 2008).

MSF began tackling the disease in the 1980s. Now, two decades later, the organization treats as many as 20% to 30%

of all sleeping sickness cases—46,200 patients in 2006 alone. Thanks to its experience in a number of high-prevalence contexts, MSF understands the challenges of managing sleeping sickness, and is working to bring innovation in three areas. The first is treatment, where existing drugs are hard to handle, often very toxic, resistance-prone, and prohibitively expensive—in the rare instances they are available. The second is diagnostic tools, which are virtually non-existent. The third is the overall operational organization of care. As we will see, MSF has been a driving force in designing disease-control policies, as well as diagnostic and therapeutic techniques. All of these efforts aim to respond to the urgent need for care.

Sleeping Sickness Wakes Up: Neglected Populations and Neglected Diseases

Sleeping sickness is a vector-borne parasitic disease that exists exclusively in sub-Saharan Africa, with the vast majority of cases in rural areas. The parasite, a protozoan of the genus *Trypanosoma (brucei gambiense),* is transmitted to man by the bite of a tsetse fly previously infected by biting human or other animal carriers of the pathogen. There is a second form, *Trypanosoma brucei rhodesiense,* but it has low prevalence in humans, progresses more rapidly, and is easier to diagnose.

The disease is characterized by an indolent, progressive course in two stages. During the first, or hemolymphatic, stage, besides posterior cervical lymphadenopathy, the clinical signs are non-specific: recurrent fever, pain, fatigue, itching. The second, or meningoencephalitic, stage, affects the central nervous system, causing pain and severe psychiatric and neurological problems. Without treatment, the disease is invariably fatal after a period of wasting and coma.

By the 1980s and 1990s—nearly a century after the first efforts to control the disease—the practical problems had changed very little. Diagnosis was complicated, and treatments such as suramin and pentamidine were only effective in stage 1 of the disease. There were only two drugs approved for stage 2: melarsoprol, which is extremely toxic, and eflornithine, which is extremely expensive.

In 1978 some research progress was made, including the creation of the Card Agglutination Test for Trypanosomiasis (CATT), while capillary tube centrifugation was already available.[1] Yet only two new drugs have been discovered in the past fifty years: eflornithine and nifurtimox. Due primarily to a lack of political will, innovations could barely get past the invention stage. "While a 'white elephant' for which no one has any use might be a great invention in terms of technological achievement, it may never become an innovation if there is no demand for it. … It's clear that a policy to stimulate technology is therefore not the same thing as a policy to develop innovation" (Blondel, 2002, p. 135). There were few actors in the field to take advantage of these developments, and the World Health Organization (WHO) had only two specialists working on the issue at the time.

In response to the resurgence of sleeping sickness, the Thirty-sixth World Health Assembly adopted resolution WHA36.31 in 1983, urging the WHO to increase controls, and a sleeping sickness prevention and control program was created the following year.

In 1992 the WHO proposed an "Initiative for Central Africa" aimed at coordinating and strengthening sleeping sickness control in the region. The project, a joint effort by the WHO, the Food and Agriculture Organization, the International Atomic Energy Agency (IAEA),[2] and the Organization of African Unity

---

1   Capillary tube centrifugation is a laboratory technique in which a small cylinder, filled by capillary action with a biological fluid, is placed into a machine that uses centrifugal force to separate sediment to be used for laboratory measurements.

2   The IAEA participates in vector control by using radiation to sterilize male tsetse flies.

(OAU), was finally launched in 1995. Support from the French and Belgian governments, and later the European Union, helped fund a program to coordinate sleeping sickness control activities in Central and West Africa. The program increased the participation of national officials and intensified collaboration with a number of institutions, including the *Organisation de Coordination et de Coopération pour la lutte contre les Grandes Endémies*, based in Ivory Coast; the *Organisation de Coordination pour la lutte contre les Endémies en Afrique Centrale*, based in Cameroon; MSF; the *Fonds Médical Tropical*; and France's *Institut de Recherche pour le Développement*. In 1997 efforts were bolstered by the adoption of resolution WHA50.36 by the Fiftieth World Health Assembly.

Despite these developments, however, management of the disease remained sketchy, which proved that the initiatives were unsuitable. As the number of actors grew, the campaigns lost coherence and long-term vision, and there was a lack of political and organizational foresight. Some believed that the focus should have been on preventing the disease from being forgotten or neglected (Jannin, 2000). Because sleeping sickness sufferers were of little economic interest, the disease was still not a priority. The combination of a neglected disease and a neglected population turned out to be particularly devastating in the affected regions (Jannin, Simarro, Louis, 2003).

In 1999 the WHO launched an international campaign to promote the control of sleeping sickness. The same year, at MSF's urging, a group of experts was formed under United Nations coordination. It issued two recommendations. First, it stressed the importance of investing in research for new drugs to treat the disease. Second, because the short- and medium-term results from this type of research are unpredictable, the experts recommended that combinations of existing drugs[3]

---

3   In 2000 Epicentre and MSF-France developed the first protocol for a combination therapy study in Uganda.

also be studied. This was when public-private partnerships were formed, and pharmaceutical firms such as Aventis, Bayer, and Bristol-Myers Squibb (BMS) joined the WHO in the fight against sleeping sickness.

In July 2000 the Pan-African Trypanosomiasis and Tsetse Eradication Campaign (PATTEC) was launched at the OAU's Summit of Heads of State and Government in Lomé. PATTEC concentrated its efforts on preparing a major anti-vector campaign, in combination with an effort to improve disease surveillance and treatment. It also worked to encourage the development of new alternatives to resistance-prone drugs.

MSF co-founded and launched the Drugs for Neglected Diseases Initiative (DNDi) in 2003, an independent, non-profit drug research and development foundation. Sleeping sickness was one of its top priorities.[4]

DNDi has focused its efforts on identifying promising new drugs, and hopes to begin clinical trials for one of them—fexinidazole. Since 2005, it has also been part of the Nifurtimox Eflornithine Combination Therapy (NECT) study, launched by Epicentre and MSF-Holland in 2003.

DNDi also set up an R&D network with academic research groups at Japan's Kitasato Institute, to develop two new clinical trial–ready drug candidates. Sleeping sickness control programs and researchers from endemic countries are also involved in these efforts (DNDi, November 2007).

From One Empirical Approach to Another: The Return of Dr. Jamot

MSF opened its first trypanosomiasis program in 1986, in the Moyo district of northern Uganda, and the teams faced the problem of how to manage the disease. This meant applying

---

4   For more on DNDi missions, see the study by C. Vidal and J. Pinel in this volume.

practices introduced by military doctors in the first half of the twentieth century.

The heart of Eugène Jamot's[5] strategy was mobile medicine and mass treatment. He increased the number of men and equipment in his teams, and sent them into the bush to screen for the disease and treat sufferers (Louis, Simarro, Lucas, 2002, p. 334). These principles, which would live on after him, involved systematic testing of all populations and a standardized regimen of diagnosis and immediate treatment. In order to succeed, Jamot developed a vertical strategy (devoted specifically to sleeping sickness) in high-prevalence areas.

When launching its sleeping sickness activities in Uganda in 1986, MSF found itself at a loss; with a lack of data, tools, and general interest, the teams were in an almost amateur situation. Epicentre[6] hadn't yet been created, and it would be another nine years (1995) before MSF-Belgium would start a similar project. Having to overcome an unwillingness (both inside and outside MSF) to challenge outdated practices only made matters worse. Initially, the disease control strategy consisted in identifying large foci of infection that were priority zones for intervention. A mobile approach was only adopted later, thanks to information from local actors as foci were discovered. So micro-epidemiology supplanted macro-epidemiology, and the practice of targeting according to previous endemic episodes was dropped. The field teams drew a map of the disease and identified high-risk areas. In the early 1980s, some Ugandans had taken refuge in tsetse fly–infested parts of Sudan. They subsequently resettled in Uganda, in regions that were also infested by the vector. Once maps were drawn up using data

---

5   Military doctor Eugène Jamot (1879–1937) developed a large-scale method for treating trypanosomiasis (Milleliri, 2004). He helped create the *Service General Autonome de la Maladie du Sommeil* in French West Africa and in Togo.

6   Epicentre is an MSF satellite organization specializing in intervention epidemiology research.

on tsetse fly prevalence in these regions (obtained from vector control agencies), disease prevalence in the Sudanese migration zones, and the origin of patients, a more rational targeting of populations became possible.

On the operational level, in addition to the vertical approach, the teams set up a system of standardized patient cards that enabled them to monitor individual patients more closely and therefore analyze actions. Later, in 1994, Epicentre developed the Epitryp electronic database, which automated mapping and medical monitoring. This tool is still being used by MSF in the field. Monitoring entire patient cohorts allowed measuring the efficacy of treatment for the first time, and confirmed what practitioners already suspected regarding the dangers of melarsoprol, at a time when an alternative like eflornithine was already known. Practitioners also noted inconsistencies between their clinical observations in Uganda and the standard disease descriptions, and challenged the criteria for determining the disease stage (Dumas and Bouteille, 2002). Their clinical and biological data were used to create the first reliable screening and diagnosis algorithms, later adopted by other medical actors (Paquet, Castilla, Mbulamberi, et al., 1995).

Laboratory diagnosis at that time was pitiful and only the erythrocyte sedimentation rate was used. At the Antwerp Institute of Tropical Medicine, Magnus, Vervoort, and Van Meirvenne had developed a new test in 1978, the CATT. It had not yet been tested *in vivo* so an application to validate the tool was needed. In 1986–87, MSF embarked on a study of the test's sensitivity and specificity. Epicentre then worked on the problem of how to interpret the results in previously treated patients with persistent antibodies (Paquet, Ancelle, Gastellu-Etchegorry, et al., 1992). Even now, the CATT does not have reliable sensitivity or specificity, and the accompanying microscopic examination is both laborious and insensitive, hence the large number of undetected cases. Moreover, the lack of adequate infrastructure makes the tests—which use molecular markers—difficult to use in rural endemic areas.

Determining the stages of the disease also remains an issue. The process involves analyzing cerebrospinal fluid in order to choose the appropriate treatment. This requires performing lumbar puncture, an invasive procedure that further complicates the diagnostic process. Better, simpler, more robust tests capable of determining the stage of the disease would revolutionize sleeping sickness control, making mass screening a more realistic objective.[7]

The effectiveness in treating large endemic foci and a larger number of dispersed low-prevalence areas changed the epidemiological landscape, requiring new approaches that were less restrictive in terms of resources, and easier to implement.

In 2004, MSF-Holland launched a pilot strategy in the Congo Republic, nicknamed "Hit and Run," based on observations: first, the limited number of programs using the eflornithine-based protocol for first-line treatment; and second, the fairly general reduction in prevalence in the region. Neither conventional programs nor active screening made sense anymore. What was needed was diagnosis and treatment at peripheral health posts, and rapid intervention in zones where cases were occurring. Using a horizontal approach integrated at the primary care level, these peripheral posts would provide passive screening and treatment. If several cases were detected from the same region, suggesting elevated prevalence in a localized area, a mobile team was sent to do active screening and on-the-spot treatment. The goal was to eliminate the disease at the source,

---

7   Laboratory diagnosis is still a major issue. Thanks to a donation from the Gates Foundation, the WHO and the Foundation for Innovative New Diagnostics have created a partnership to develop and assess new tests that are simpler, more accurate, and less expensive than existing ones.

even if this meant not fully eradicating it. The positive results obtained with this strategy led MSF to create and distribute a standard protocol for its field programs in endemic areas.

Monotherapy: Unorthodox Alliances

In the early twentieth century, the first sleeping sickness treatment protocols used an arsenic derivative called atoxyl. A compound from the same family, melarsoprol, is still being used today. After tryparsamide was synthesized in the early 1920s, and the number of treatment failures grew, various arsenic-based combination therapies were tested. At the same time, non-arsenic-based medications such as pentamidine were developed in the 1940s and adopted for use in mass prophylaxis campaigns (Ollivier, Legros, 2001). There was a lot of inertia and very little originality in the development of new and effective drugs in the 1980s. Melarsoprol had devastating side effects, and eflornithine—a very promising drug synthesized in 1979—was still little known, in limited production, expensive, and required significant human and financial resources for poor countries. Nifurtimox, used for the first time in 1980, was not yet being considered for treatment of sleeping sickness because phase 2 and phase 3 clinical trials were needed to confirm its effects.[8]

Proving the Efficacy or Inefficacy of Existing Drugs

Studies on trypanosome's melarsoprol resistance were the starting point for MSF's recent innovations for treating stage 2 of the disease.

In 1949, Friedheim developed the organic arsenical melar-

---

8   Nifurtimox is a drug prescribed for treatment of Chagas disease. It has been used off-label for treating sleeping sickness, particularly in Zaire and Sudan in the 1980s. Cheap and easy to use, promising in combination, it appears to be better tolerated than melarsoprol, despite some side effects, which include anorexia, weight loss, and neurological effects. A donation of nifurtimox for use in treatment of sleeping sickness was obtained through a 2004 agreement between Bayer and the WHO. This medication was intended for clinical trials and for compassionate use, usually off-label, as an alternative to eflornithine in melarsoprol failure.

soprol (or Mel B), an atoxyl derivative whose advantage is that it lacks tryparsamide's potential for optic nerve toxicity. As the standard treatment for stage 2, it helps—at least partially—with the problem of arsenic resistance, but at the cost of deadly arsenic-related encephalopathies (5% to 10%). It also has to be administered under direct medical supervision in a hospital. Intravenous administration and toxicity therefore limit its use in everyday practice, particularly by mobile treatment teams. MSF quickly discovered the limits of using this standard drug in the field. A follow-up analysis in 1994 on the seven thousand patients included in the program since 1986 in Uganda added to fears about melarsoprol use.[9] In 1992 and 1993 there were two outbreaks of post-treatment reactive encephalopathy at the sleeping sickness treatment center in Adjumani, during which more than 10% of patients treated with melarsoprol developed arsenical encephalopathy. Retrospective studies helped identify exogenous risk factors—in particular, concurrent use of an anti-parasitic agent (thiabendazole) and poor general health at the start of treatment (Ancelle et al., 1994). A few years later, Epicentre published the first study showing an increased failure rate with melarsoprol in the Omugo program in northern Uganda. While the expected rate was usually between 3% and 9%, the study revealed that nearly 30% of the 428 patients treated from 1995 to 1997 were in treatment failure (Legros, Fournier, Gastellu-Etchegorry, et al., 1999a; Legros et al., 1999b).

In paediatrics, a retrospective case study of children under six years old treated in an MSF sleeping sickness treatment center in southern Sudan between 2000 and 2002 showed that clinical signs alone were not adequate for determining the stage of the disease. Laboratory staging was therefore essential to avoid the unnecessary use of melarsoprol, with its adverse effects (Eperon et al., 2007). In addition, melarsoprol was just

---

9   Epicentre set up a permanent base in Uganda to help MSF projects with their research and innovation efforts.

as toxic in this age group, making first-line use of eflornithine absolutely necessary in both children and adults.

Ultimately, melarsoprol resistance—brought to light in 1999—was a major argument for prioritizing research for stage 2 sleeping sickness treatments. The scientific community and pharmaceutical companies failed to heed the call, however, so MSF began looking for alternatives. This included making better use of drugs already on the market—hence the interest in eflornithine.

Also known as DFMO or Ornidyl, eflornithine is an anti-mitotic agent approved for the treatment of cancer. Its anti-protozoal properties in late-stage sleeping sickness were confirmed by Bacchi and his team in the 1980s (Bacchi, Nathan, Hutner, et al., 1980; McCann, Bacchi, Clarkson, et al., 1981). Van Nieuwenhove put it to the test in southern Sudan, where about twenty sleeping sickness patients—eighteen of them in stage 2 and sixteen of them arsenical-resistant—received oral eflornithine monotherapy (Van Nieuwenhove, Schechter, Declercq, et al., 1985). Soon after the study's publication in 1990, the drug was approved for this indication by the US Food and Drug Administration.

Eflornithine's advantage lay in its relative lack of toxicity compared to melarsoprol and its efficacy in arsenical-resistant patients. It was, however, very complex to use (four infusions a day for fourteen days) and too expensive for African populations, and so it went out of production in 1995.

In early 2000 there was little in scientific literature about eflornithine. The few studies being done showed a near-absence of the encephalopathies observed with melarsoprol, but a substantial mortality rate of between 2% and 6%. A series of studies in Africa was therefore needed to confirm expectations for the drug. That year, MSF-France took over a trypanosomiasis program that had been started by MSF-Holland in Ibba, Sudan, in 1999. After just over a year, the epidemiological surveillance system in the remote, conflict-ridden area revealed worrying melarsoprol failure rates of around 30%. Because eflornithine was not available, MSF began using a new protocol combining melarsoprol and nifurtimox. In September 2001, however—thanks to a drug donation from Aventis and Sudanese government authorization and involvement—eflornithine was adopted for first-line, fourteen-day monotherapy. This illustrates the fundamental role played by the authorities in MSF-intervention countries in the implementation, follow-up, and success of studies. Ibba became the first project in Africa to use eflornithine as the first-line treatment for stage 2 sleeping sickness—despite the objections of some within MSF, who felt there was not enough evidence to support using this protocol.

The results were positive: 1% mortality in the first cohort, then 1.2% in larger cohorts, with a drug that was well tolerated and effective (Priotto, 2008). At the same time, it appeared that the quality of nursing care played a crucial role in the treatment. Indeed, the results for the first Ibba cohort showed that mortality could be attributed, in part, to infections due to poor infusion techniques. Improvements in nursing care helped make the use of eflornithine safer.

MSF-Switzerland also had a program in southern Sudan, which started in 2000 in Kajo-Keji. The results from Ibba justified introducing eflornithine as the first-line treatment there in January 2003. The protocol change was a success. A retrospective comparison between the melarsoprol cohort (June 2000 to December 2002, n = 708) and the eflornithine cohort (January 2003 to December 2003, n = 251) showed a significant difference in mortality during treatment (3.5% for melarsoprol, versus 0.8% for eflornithine), and no difference in mortality or relapse rates at twelve months post-treatment.

Several recommendations resulted from this study: first, that eflornithine be the drug of choice for stage 2 of the disease, not just in areas of high melarsoprol resistance; and second, that research on combination therapies be undertaken to minimize the emergence of resistance (Chappuis et al., 2005).[10]

Making Eflornithine Available

In 1995, it was announced that eflornithine would no longer be produced, due to its prohibitive cost for African countries.

The company that made eflornithine—in the midst of a merger with Hoechst—was selling the anti-parasitic at cost price. Not making any profit, it granted licensing rights for the drug to the WHO, which would have to find another company to manufacture it. Though dozens of drug companies were contacted, none offered to do it at a low enough price. Only the original manufacturer—which had by then become Aventis—was willing to provide the WHO and MSF with a limited and irregular supply, until the inventory on hand was exhausted.

In the field, lots were delivered sparingly for clinical trials or for compassionate use in melarsoprol failure. In 1999, MSF received one of Aventis' last ad hoc donations—ten thousand ampoules of eflornithine from the 1995 production (they had been used to treat relapses in Uganda). Jean Jannin of the WHO then confirmed that "the situation was becoming downright worrying. It was obvious that eflornithine would run out before the end of 2001. The situation for other treatments wasn't much better. Whether intended for the early stage of the disease (pentamidine and suramin) or the late stage (melarsoprol and nifurtimox), all drugs were more or less in danger of running out.

---

10   The Republic of Congo also provided fertile ground for progress on sleeping sickness. A retrospective study using data collected on the Gamboma, Bouenza, and Mossaka programs (MSF-Holland) from 2001 to 2005 confirmed earlier results and lent strength to the idea that eflornithine was less toxic and more effective than melarsoprol. The authors then recommended eflornithine as the first-line treatment in the Republic of Congo.

Bayer and Aventis weren't sure whether they would continue production" (*Libération*, February 21, 2001).

MSF considered having the drug manufactured, but it was a complex process, beyond the scope of the organization's expertise. As it turned out, production was rescued by an eflornithine-based depilatory cream marketed by BMS under the name *Vaniqa*. MSF and the Campaign for Access to Essential Medicines then joined forces to create a lobbying group, and approach Aventis and BMS, while pushing the WHO to shoulder the responsibility.

On May 3, 2001, after two years of talks, MSF, Aventis, Bayer, and other private partners established with the WHO a public-private partnership to fight sleeping sickness. Aventis signed a $25 million, five-year donation agreement (2001–2006). This collaboration agreement with the WHO had three components:

- Drug donation: the company pledged to produce and supply eflornithine, melarsoprol, and pentamidine free of charge.[11] Storage, distribution, and delivery of the donated drugs would be the responsibility of MSF-Logistique in Merignac, which would be managing the stock for all prescribers worldwide. All orders from national programs and NGOs would need prior WHO approval. When the agreement ended in 2006, Aventis said they wanted to transfer the technology to another pharmaceutical company, if one would agree to continue production (Prescrire, 2006).
- Surveillance and control: with agreed financial backing from Aventis, the WHO pledged to speed up disease control activities by supporting national programs, in particular for training medical personnel and routine screening in endemic zones.

---

11 *Sleeping Sickness. MSF Fact Sheet*, MSF and the Campaign for Access to Essential Medicines, May 2004.

- Research and development: financial support was also intended to help organize new research via the WHO's Program for Research and Training in Tropical Diseases (TDR),[12] with an emphasis on adapting treatments, developing new methods for making one of the existing products and, ultimately, developing new drugs.

In agreement with Aventis, BMS promised to finance a one-year supply (60,000 vials) of eflornithine's active ingredient, and pledged $400,000 over two years to the WHO to support treatment efforts. In 2002, Bayer agreed to supply as much suramin as the WHO felt necessary, free of charge, for five years. At the same time, the company supported studies on the use of nifurtimox for treating sleeping sickness.

A WHO press release on the Aventis–WHO agreement cited MSF's central role: "Both WHO and Aventis commend non-governmental organizations, especially MSF, for the public awareness raised on sleeping sickness affecting poor African countries" (WHO, 2001). What made these alliances unique was the crossing of interests between, on the one hand, humanitarian organizations, concerned with the urgent need for treatment, and, on the other, companies, concerned about their corporate image. Within MSF, the strategy was a delicate balance between opportunism and risk-taking, not to mention the ambiguity of simultaneously challenging and collaborating with pharmaceutical firms.

In 2006, Sanofi Aventis and the WHO signed a new agreement extending the five-year agreement signed in 2001.[13]

---

12   Supported by the United Nations Children's Fund, the United Nations Development Programme, the World Bank, and the WHO.

13   The terms of the earlier agreement regarding the production and donation of drugs (pentamidine, melarsoprol, and eflornithine) were renewed, in addition to a $5 million donation. Again, there was an additional financial contribution of $20 million to fight the four most neglected tropical diseases (trypanosomiasis, leishmaniasis, Buruli ulcer, and Chagas disease).

Simplifying Treatment Delivery to Patients

In 2006—five years after free access, and before the WHO–Sanofi Aventis agreement was renewed—only 20% of patients were getting first-line eflornithine. These were primarily the patients treated by MSF. Simplified distribution and a free supply of the infusions and other solutions needed by national programs to implement the protocol were essential. The DFMO (eflornithine) kit was therefore created, and presented by MSF to the 28th Meeting of the International Scientific Council for Trypanosomiasis Research and Control (ISCTRC)[14] in Addis Ababa in 2005. The WHO and MSF-Logistique worked together to create the kits, which were ready in 2007. The 2006 Sanofi–WHO agreement ensured that production and supply would be free (to the capitals of requesting countries).

Combination Therapies: Daring Clinical Trials

It is currently believed that it will be more than ten years before there is a new drug for treating stage 2 sleeping sickness. In the meantime, drug combinations, which are easier to administer and require smaller doses and a shorter course of treatment, are considered the best way to meet patient needs. They also provide relative protection against resistance.

As early as 1998, a WHO technical report judged it "essential that the possibility of drug combinations be thoroughly explored" (WHO, 1998) and, in 1999, the Human African Trypanosomiasis Treatment and Drug Resistance Network, to which MSF belonged, identified combination therapies, including nifurtimox, as one of its research priorities (WHO, 2001). It was also at this time that the internal MSF sleeping sickness working group was created. The group's purpose was to highlight priorities in sleeping sickness treatment, centralize

---

14 The ISCTRC is a statutory body of the African Union; it meets every two years.

information coming from different field projects, and harmonize recommendations.

In early 2001 the first MSF patients were enrolled in the three bi-therapy trials at the Omugo site in Uganda. This was a comparative trial, in which patients were randomly allocated to three groups for the three possible combinations (nifurtimox-eflornithine, nifurtimox-melarsoprol, and eflornithine-melarsoprol). This first study, highly exploratory in design, proposed starting directly in phase 3, thereby bypassing the pre-clinical and clinical phases 1 and 2, which would have required an enormous amount of funding. The new protocol proposed four injections per day of eflornithine, but for only one week instead of two, and ten days of nifurtimox instead of thirty. The study began in 2001, but soon had to be stopped because two of the groups turned out to be toxic, with four deaths in the melarsoprol-nifurtimox group and one death in the melarsoprol-eflornithine group. There was also a significant drop in prevalence.[15] Not enough patients could be recruited to provide conclusive statistics for the otherwise encouraging nifurtimox-eflornithine group (Priotto et al., 2006).

To remedy this situation, the Nifurtimox-Eflornithine Case Series study was launched at MSF's Yumbé site in Uganda in 2002.

The results of the two studies were unprecedented: a 100% cure rate for the nifurtimox-eflornithine combination, with no deaths or relapses at two years—but the sample size was still considered inadequate to confirm these conclusions.

The NECT study protocol was written by Epicentre in 2002 in collaboration with an international scientific committee. It proposed comparing nifurtimox-eflornithine to eflornithine

---

15   The MSF project was already showing good results by the time the Epicentre study got underway!

alone. The aim was to prove that the combination of these two drugs was as safe and effective as eflornithine monotherapy and also easier to use. The study design was based on these constraints. It contained three important changes: the combination of eflornithine with nifurtimox, a reduction in the number of daily infusions from four to two while keeping the total daily dose the same, and a shorter duration of treatment, from fourteen days to seven. It was not yet known how the drugs would react in combination.

There was some opposition, at the WHO in particular, but also within MSF and DNDi. The study was delayed for a while for lack of nifurtimox, which the WHO refused to supply, citing, on one hand, the lack of knowledge about its effects (research on which dates back to the mid-twentieth century), and, on the other, the failure to respect biomedical ethics and to conform to usual clinical trial standards—a conflict reminiscent of the 1990s epistemic crisis in the research world (Dodier, Barbot, 2000). There is still some debate over the benefits and limitations of the *Guidelines for Good Clinical Practice* (ICH, 1996),[16] which affect research in general, especially into tropical diseases in the developing world (White, 2006). As with the ACT UP model for AIDS in the 1980s, the urgency of finding answers justified taking risks and ignoring standard rules in the development of new treatments. Epicentre and MSF adapted their practices and GCPs to suit the intervention context, while preserving the basic ethical and methodological rules related to safety and patient consent.

The NECT study began in 2003 in a trypanosomiasis control program run by MSF-Holland at the Nkayi site in the Congo Republic, thanks to a specific nifurtimox donation by Bayer. Unfortunately, supply and authorization problems meant the

16 GCPs are rules written and imposed by industrialized nations to prevent scientific fraud, improve documentation, and ensure respect for the Declaration of Helsinki (1964), which protects the rights of patients participating in clinical trials.

program got off to a late start, and after more than a year and a half of recruitment efforts, the sample size was still too small to complete the study.

The study required a sample size of 280 patients, which implied a multi-center study. Epicentre decided to explore other operational sites, and came to an agreement with MSF-Belgium, which in 2004 was preparing to open a project in the Democratic Republic of Congo (DRC). The two main opponents to these trials, DNDi and WHO–TDR, joined the study in 2005.

Without the experience in Nkayi, it is likely that the multi-center study would have been delayed for another four or five years because of the strict standard recommendations. MSF and Epicentre decided to risk using the NECT protocol, relying on the initial results to convince skeptics that the trials should progress much more quickly.

The study became multi-centric, with three major sponsors: MSF-Holland, DNDi, and the WHO's TDR program. The TDR-funded sites later withdrew, however, and Epicentre's analysis included only the results from the other four.

The study at the first center, launched at the Nkayi site in 2003 by MSF, has ended. The combination is better tolerated than eflornithine alone, and its non-inferiority has held so far (two relapses in each group). The hospitalization stages for the other three sites in the DRC ended in late 2006, and there will be analyses on patient follow-up. This trial is undoubtedly an innovation in the treatment of stage 2 sleeping sickness (Priotto et al., 2009). Compared to eflornithine alone, the eflornithine-nifurtimox combination is easier to use, less expensive, and less toxic (it causes less neutropenia, thus reducing the risk of infection).

Since 2004 MSF has been treating 20% to 30% of all sleeping sickness cases using first-line eflornithine for stage 2 of the disease in all its programs. With the introduction of the DFMO (eflornithine) kits, there is a realistic hope that more cases in Africa will be treated using this protocol. MSF had made a crucial contribution in research and innovation by accurately and systematically documenting its experiences, and by publishing and presenting its results in international forums. MSF has institutional expertise and responsibility with regard to sleeping sickness, making it one of the foremost authorities on medical treatment of the disease. Vector control, on the other hand, is not one of its strong points.

Sleeping sickness prevalence remains high in the DRC, Angola, and southern Sudan. MSF, Epicentre, DNDi, and the WHO are collaborating in the fight against trypanosomiasis, working together to help health ministries in the affected countries draft protocols and other guidelines, as well as train care providers and technical staff. The difficulty MSF now faces lies with its operational choices. There is a need to consolidate knowledge, but the drop in prevalence and the replacement of large foci by scattered, smaller foci means that intervention by specialized MSF programs can no longer be justified.

A medium-term commitment, for example with a national or trans-national mobile team capable of responding to alerts from different endemic zones, is one possibility; in any case, the therapeutic innovations from the NECT trial will appear all the more pertinent when applied in the field. A massive effort will be needed to get this protocol recommended as the first-line therapy.

Bibliography

Ancelle, T., B. Barret, L. Flachet, A. Moren. 1994. "Étude de deux épidémies d'encéphalopathies arsénicales dans le traitement de la trypanosomiase, Uganda, 1992–1993." *Bulletin de la Société de Pathologie Exotique* 87 (5): 341–346.

Bacchi, C. J., H. C. Nathan, S. H. Hutner, et al. 1980. "Polyamine metabolism: a potential therapeutic target in trypanosomes." *Science* 210 (4467): 332–334.

Blondel, D. 2002. "Le rôle des scientifiques dans le processus d'innovation." In N. Altrer, editor, *Les logiques de l'innovation*. Paris: La Découverte&Syros.

Cattand, P. 2001. "L'épidémiologie de la trypanosomiase humaine africaine: une histoire multifactorielle complexe." *Médecine Tropicale* 61 (4-5): 313–322.

Chappuis, F., N. Udayraj, K. Steitenroth, A. Meussen, P.A. Bovieret. 2005. Eflornithine is Safer than Melarsoprol for the Treatment of Second-Stage Trypanosoma brucei gambiense Human African Trypanosomiasis." *Clinical Infectious Diseases* 41 (5): 748–751.

Courtin, F., V. Jamonneau, G. Duvallet, A. Garcia, B. Coulibaly, J.P. Doumenge, G. Cuny, P. Solano. 2008. "Sleeping sickness in West Africa (1906–2006): changes in spatial repartition and lessons from the past." *Tropical Medicine & International Health* 13 (3): 334–344.

Dodier, N., J. Barbot. 2000. "Le temps des tensions épistémiques: le développement des essais thérapeutiques dans le cadre du sida." *Revue française de Sociologie* 41 (1): 79–118.

Drugs for Neglected Diseases Initiative. 2006. *DNDi newsletter*. No. 14. http://www.dndi.org/newsletters/n14/page1.htm.

Dumas, M., B. Bouteille. 2002. "La trypanosomose humaine africaine: propos sur le traitement actuel et les perspectives." *Bulletin de la Société de Pathologie Exotique* 95 (5): 341–344.

Eperon, G., C. Schmid, L. Loutan, F. Chappuis. 2007. "Clinical presentation and treatment outcome of sleeping sickness in Sudanese pre-school children." *Acta Tropica* 101 (1): 31–39.

Hamel, A. 2001. "Genèse de la Campagne pour l'Accès aux Médicaments Essentiels." *Humanitaire* 3: 115–123.

International Conference on Harmonisation of Technical Requirements for Registration of Pharmaceuticals for Human Use. 1996. *ICH Harmonised Tripartite Guideline. Guideline for Good Clinical Practice.* Current Step 4 version.

Jannin, J. 2000. "Actualités de la trypanosomiase humaine." *Médecine Tropicale* 60 (2S): 56–57.

Jannin, J., P. P. Simarro, F. J. Louis. 2003. "Le concept de maladie négligée." *Médecine Tropicale* 63 (3): 219–221.

Legros, D., C. Fournier, M. Gastellu-Etchegorry, F. Maiso, E. Szumilin. 1999a. "Échecs thérapeutiques du mélarsoprol parmi des patients traités au stade tardif de trypanosomose humaine africaine à T. b. gambiense en Ouganda." *Bulletin de la Société de Pathologie* Exotique 92 (3): 171–172.

Legros, D., S. Evans, F. Maiso, J.C Enyaru, D. Mbulamberi. 1999b. "Risk factors for treatment failure after melarsoprol for Trypanosoma brucei gambiense trypanosomiasis in Uganda." *Transactions of the Royal Society of Tropical Medicine and Hygiene* 93 (4): 439–442.

Louis, F. J., P. P. Simarro, P. Lucas. 2002. "Maladie du sommeil: cent ans d'évolution des stratégies de lutte." *Bulletin de la Société de Pathologie Exotique* 95 (5): 331–336.

McCann, P.P., C.J. Bacchi, A.B. Clarkson, J.R Seed, H.C Nathan, B.O. Amole, S.H. Hunter, A. Sjoerdsma. 1981. "Further studies on difluoromethylornithine in African trypanosomes." *Medical Biology* 59 (5–6): 434–40.

Milleliri, J.-M. 2004. "Jamot, cet inconnu." *Bulletin de la Société de Pathologie Exotique* 97 (3): 213–222.

Olivier, G., D. Legros. 2001. "Trypanosomiase humaine africaine: historique de la thérapeutique et de ses échecs." *Tropical Medicine and International Health* 6 (11): 855–863.

Paquet C., T. Ancelle, M. Gastellu-Etchegorry, J. Castilla, I. Harndt. 1992. "Persistence of antibodies to Trypanosoma brucei gambiense after treatment of human trypanosomiasis in Uganda." *The Lancet* 340 (8813): 250.

Paquet C., J. Castilla, D. Mbulamberi, M.F. Beaulieu, M. Gastellu-Etchegorry, A. Moren. 1995. "La trypanosomiase à Trypanosoma brucei gambiense dans le foyer du Nord-Ouest de l'Ouganda. Bilan de 5 années de lutte (1987–1991)." *Bulletin de la Société de Pathologie Exotique* 88 (1): 38–41.

Prescrire. 2006. "Editorial. Maladie du sommeil: la cosmétologie au secours de la santé publique." *Prescrire* 26 (269): 135–136.

Priotto G., C. Fogg, M. Balasegaram, O. Erphas, A. Louga, F. Checci, S. Ghabri, P. Piola. 2006. "Three Drug Combinations for Late-Stage *Trypanosoma brucei gambiense* Sleeping Sickness: A Randomised Clinical Trial in Uganda." doi:10.1371/journal.pctr.0010039. PLoS *Clinical Trials* 1 (8): e39.

Priotto G., L. Pinoges, I. B. Fursa, B. Burke, N. Nicolay, G. Grillet, C. Hewison, M. Balasegaram. 2008. "Safety and effectiveness of first line eflornithine for *Trypanosoma brucei gambiense* sleeping sickness in Sudan: cohort study." doi:10.1136/bmj.39485.592674. BE. *British Medical Journal* 336: 705–708,

Priotto G., S. Kasparian, W. Mutombo, D. Ngouama, S. Ghorashian. 2009. "Multicentre randomised non-inferiority trial of nifurtimox-eflornithine combination therapy for second-stage gambiense sleeping sickness." *The Lancet* 374 (9683): 56–64.

Van Nieuwenhove S., P. J. Schechter, J. Declercq, G. Bone, J. Burke, A. Sjoerdsma. 1985. "Treatment of gambiense sleeping sickness in the Sudan with oral DFMO (DL-alpha-difluoromethylornithine), an inhibitor of ornithine decarboxylase; first field trial." *Transactions of the Royal Society of Tropical Medicine and Hygiene* 79 (5): 692–698.

World Health Organization (WHO). 1998. *Control and Surveillance of African Trypanosomiasis. Report of a WHO Expert Committee*, Technical Report Series 881. Geneva: World Health Organization.

——. 2001a. "World Health Organization and Aventis Announce a Major Initiative to Step Up Efforts Against Sleeping Sickness." Press release. 3 May. Geneva.

——. 2001b. *HAT Treatment and Drug Resistance Network. Report of the Second and Third Steering Committee Meetings. 29 September 1999, Mombasa, Kenya; 28–30 May 2000, Bruges, Belgium*, WHO/CDS/CSR/EDC/2001.13.

White, N. J. 2006. "Editorial. Clinical trials in tropical diseases: a politically incorrect view." *Tropical Medicine & International Health* 11 (10): 1483–1484.

Chapter 8

Malaria

Introducing ACT from Asia to Africa

Suna Balkan and Jean-François Corty

Nearly one million deaths are attributed to malaria each year (World Health Organization (WHO), 2008), 91% in Africa and 85% in children less than five years of age. Although these figures are biased by inadequate national statistics, they do give some idea of the effect of parasitic infections due to plasmodiae species (*falciparum*, *malariae*, *ovale*, and *vivax*) (Snow, 2004). Malaria is common throughout the inter-tropical zone, and in reality may infect five hundred million people, and kill between two and three million people a year. Over one hundred countries and half of the world's population live under threat of this febrile illness, of which some forms (principally *Plasmodium falciparum*) can lead to death, and is a major cause of infectious disease mortality. Current recommendations to reduce morbidity and mortality are based on the use of insecticides (house spraying and mosquito net impregnation), intermittent prophylaxis for pregnant women, biological confirmation of disease diagnosis, and treatment with Artemisinin-based Combination Therapy (ACT). The disease's effect on health and survival rates in African children is proof that these recommendations are not properly implemented on the continent. At the end of the 1990s there were neither biological tests nor effective treatment in public health structures in many sub-Saharan African countries, leading to the development of resistance to standard therapies.

155

The efficacy of quinine, an alkaloid extracted from the bark of the quinquina tree, has been known since 1630. In 1944 Robert Woodward and William Doering from Harvard University published an article describing its complete chemical synthesis—then relatively laborious and costly compared to the technique of purifying natural quinine in use at the time. The technique proved useful during the Second World War when allied troops experienced quinine shortages. Later, in the 1950s and 1960s, the fight against malaria concentrated on vector reduction. The strategy was based on the eradication of the anopheles mosquito vector for interhuman transmission in defined areas, notably in Africa, using an insecticide, DDT. Despite initial successes, the use of DDT declined following the appearance of resistance, information on DDT toxicity, and campaigns by environmental groups.[1]

In parallel, chloroquine (1947) and sulfadoxine-pyrimethamine (SP) (1969) were introduced for the treatment of simple forms of malaria. During the period of decolonization, antimalarial development was more a military than a public health concern for ex-colonial powers. The later wars in Asia were the starting point of intense military medical research.

During the 1960s and 1970s American medical research, stimulated by the large numbers of soldiers affected in Vietnam as well as the increasing resistance to available anti-malarials, led to the development of new molecules including halofantrine and mefloquine (MFQ). The North Vietnamese, trying to solve similar problems, turned to their Chinese allies, who proposed a family of molecules derived from artemisinin (artesunate and artemether, for example) extracted from a plant used in traditional Chinese medicine (a sagewort or wormwood, *Artemisia annua L.*). The American and Chinese discoveries came too late to influence the outcome of the conflict, but opened possibilities

---

1   Although WHO recommendations since 2007 have reintroduced the use of DDT for spraying inside houses.

for the treatment of malaria strains resistant to the preceding generation of treatments (chloroquine and SP) in Asia, Latin America, and, later, in Africa (1979). Localized resistance to MFQ and halofantrine and their side effects ended the competition between the Walter Reed Army Institute of Research and traditional Chinese medicine used by the Maoist regime. The efficacy of artemisinin derivatives and their lesser toxicity mean they were top of the list of candidates to replace older treatments that had become, or were becoming, obsolete.[2] The adoption of ACTs by national and international health authorities met with three obstacles, however: political, economic, and scientific. ACTs were the symbols of political and military defeat, and, furthermore, were developed in a scientific context outside of evidence-based medicine. Randomized clinical trials, comparing the candidate to a reference product in double-blind conditions where neither the patient nor the investigator knows which product is administered—obligatory for international recognition—had not been performed. From an economic point of view, the fact that they originated in China complicated patent applications that would have guaranteed twenty years of commercial monopoly and attracted investors. It was essential to prove that compounds including artemisinin derivatives were superior to other medications in order to change treatment protocols in response to increasing drug resistance. Scientific studies conforming to international standards were required. Furthermore, it was also necessary to find an economic model allowing African countries to guarantee supply. The introduction of rapid tests and ACTs in MSF missions, along with the plea for their accessibility in public structures in African countries, opened the way for accurate diagnosis and effective treatment. MSF's participation in their introduction through work in humanitarian circumstances (war refugees, neglected

---

2   Rapid and frequent resistance development is highly probable when monotherapies are used. It should be noted that *Plasmodium falciparum* becomes sensitive to chloroquine again after it is not used for a period of time in a given region.

epidemics) and the long mediation process (from Asia to Africa, from Chinese science to international norms, from one economic model to another, etc.) remind us that medical progress arises not only from the most sophisticated research laboratories but also from the porosity of borders and from improbable meetings between refugees, researchers, and clinicians.

The 1980s and 1990s: The Asian Experience

Refugees and Scientific Research

MSF assisted hundreds of thousands of Khmer refugees on the Thai–Cambodian border during the 1980s. On the opposing Thai–Burmese border, MSF was also caring for tens of thousands of Burmese refugees in makeshift camps in Thailand. In both cases, the inhabitants, particularly the men, regularly crossed the border into Burma or Cambodia, through malaria-infested forest zones. Population movements in militarily unstable, unhealthy frontier zones, home to informal economic activity (particularly the trade of precious stones and tropical wood), smuggling, and uncontrolled medication use, seem to have played a role in the development of poly-resistant malaria and its geographical expansion.

In these zones, MSF was confronted by a particular kind of malaria often affecting young adults in good health, and it engendered a feeling of increasing impotence. The children were protected as long as they stayed in the camps that were less infested than border forest regions. At the end of the 1980s, refugee camp doctors became worried, seeing patients returning shortly after malaria treatment with recurrent symptoms. It was these clinicians who initially suspected the development of resistance to MFQ treatment.[3]

---

3   MFQ was being prescribed as a single dose of fifteen mg/kg/day. Doubts led to several resistance studies evaluating an MFQ-Fansidar combination (called Fansimef) and different MFQ dosages as a monotherapy.

Suspicions of treatment failure based on clinical observations triggered scientific works carried out by the Shoklo Malaria Research Unit (SMRU). The SMRU, a Tropical Medicine Department field unit of Mahidol University in Bangkok, was created in 1986 in the Shoklo Burmese refugee camp (Tak province, Thailand) and led by a doctor who had previously worked on site with MSF (Nosten, 2000). It was part of the partnership between the Tropical Medicine school of Mahidol University, Bangkok, and the Oxford University Research Unit.[4] The team was mostly made up of refugees, who also occupied senior posts, and its research aimed to "benefit populations along the border, including refugees and other migrants." Relations between the SMRU and MSF were based on complementarity. The research team could not perform its work if it had to confront the refugee population's health needs single-handedly, and MSF could not adequately treat poly-resistant malaria, a major cause of camp mortality, without scientific research support. The two teams were united by a common desire to help the refugees and the shared fear of the development of untreatable malaria. Relations were dynamic despite the potential for medical, scientific, ethical, and political tensions, and for institutional rivalries. SMRU partnerships in countries influenced by China (Vietnam, Cambodia, and Burma) led to English translations of Chinese medical literature, and the consideration of the role of artemisinin derivatives in the therapeutic arsenal.

Most of the clinical studies evaluating artemisinin-derivative bi-therapy (combined with other anti-malarials) at the beginning of the 1990s were performed in the camps on the Burmese border. These products were not recommended in Thai national protocols, but were available on the market. The high number of severe malaria cases in the camps meant quality

---

4   Its principal donor is the Welcome Trust (United Kingdom).

scientific research had to be carried out to identify new treatments, and the camps' context made this research feasible. Patient follow-up was made easier by the confines of refugee camps: the number of patients lost to follow-up in studies was limited, and the medical personnel lived on site.

The first results benefited MSF patients as early as 1994. Uncomplicated malaria was treated with MFQ and artesunate, with one treatment per day for three days (Luxemburger et al., 1994). Three years later, MSF introduced artemether, an injectable artemisinin derivative, once the advantages of this treatment compared with quinine had been proven (quicker reduction in parasite load and fever and simplified administration). The Thai Health Ministry recognized the public health risk of resistance development in the refugee camps. Although the new treatment protocols had not yet been adopted nationally, their use was tolerated under certain conditions (biological confirmation of the diagnosis and regular detailed reports to provincial and national authorities).

Available classical treatments were ineffective and the last option, the treatment of uncomplicated malaria using quinine and tetracycline, was limited by adherence issues due to the need to take numerous tablets three times a day for seven days. Furthermore, quinine's side effects also caused patients to abandon treatment, and tetracycline use is not usually recommended for young children and pregnant women. The generalization of quinine for uncomplicated cases and the frequent nonadherence to a seven-day treatment protocol which also presented side effects increased the risk of quinine resistance—and quinine was the only readily available treatment for severe malaria. Other therapeutic options were urgently needed. In 1996–97, artemisinin derivative combinations were routinely prescribed as first-line therapy for uncomplicated malaria in Thai camps. Some MSF staff soon saw the potential for ACT use in sub-Saharan Africa for patients, health workers, and general public health. The question of biological confirmation of malaria diagnosis nevertheless remained a problem. According to opinions at the time, resistance development was not only due to the administration of monotherapies, but also partially due to unjustified anti-malarial prescriptions without biological confirmation of the disease.

The Need for Biological Confirmation of the Diagnosis

In Thailand in the 1990s, ACT treatment was preceded by dyed-blood microscopy (thick and thin films) to confirm diagnosis and specify the *Plasmodium* sub-species, as only *Plasmodium falciparum* malaria was associated with resistance and mortality. This prerequisite was not particularly problematic in standard local contexts involving low numbers of cases. Transmission rates were generally low, and health structures adequately supplied with staff and material. Biological confirmation could, however, be compromised by more difficult conditions such as epidemic peaks, population isolation, and population displacements. It was not always possible to perform numerous malaria smears and qualified personnel were often absent during crises. Such was the case across the border in Burma, where MSF was trying to develop activities to aid populations in significantly more resource limited settings than those in the Thai camps. A high number of malaria cases were reported; these were diagnosed too late, and were often fatal. If it were possible to confirm the diagnosis of malaria with rapid tests, artemisinin derivative therapies could be used in isolated areas as an alternative to failing MFQ monotherapy. Health authorities again tolerated the prescription of these new molecules on the condition of biological confirmation of the disease so as to avoid excessive use.

In 1996 MSF succeeded in sending mobile teams to diagnose and treat malaria cases among isolated populations in Burma that were frequently being forced to move by the army and guerrilla groups. They were also able to evaluate rapid test use in field conditions.[5]

Initial results were promising. The test was easy to use, but deteriorating security conditions and the interruption of its manufacture brought an end to the evaluation. It would be attempted once again, a few years later, in Africa.

Malaria in Africa: A Disturbing Situation

Malaria treatments varied across African countries in the 1990s, and MSF generally applied national protocols based on WHO recommendations. Chloroquine, introduced at the end of the Second World War, contained malaria transmission and reduced morbidity and mortality until the end of the 1960s. Chloroquine resistance appeared in the 1970s, however, and grew progressively, justifying a shift to SP in a few East African countries. The parasite quickly developed worrying levels of resistance to this second drug. At the beginning of the 1990s, both treatments failed regularly in children, who are at the highest risk of death from malaria. Both drugs nonetheless remained in WHO recommendations and African national protocols, as national and international authorities considered proof of their inefficacy insufficient to justify the serious consequences of change. These consequences included significant budget increases, administrative authorizations, international supply, universal distribution, and prescription training for personnel.

Also, according to opinions at the time, malaria was deemed less severe in Africa than in Asia or in South America, where resistance had developed more rapidly. Constant high transmission rates in many African countries were thought to lead to better population immunity and lower incidences of severe malaria in adults. It is undeniably simplistic, however, to ascribe a uniform

---

5   The Parasight rapid test was used to study an epidemic in the Hmong population in April 1997 (Bee Ree village).

epidemiological profile to all African countries. Malaria transmission is highly unstable in some regions, reducing population immunity and leading to severe malaria in adults, particularly pregnant women. Moreover, despite the lag in the frequency and severity of resistance development, it was above all in Africa that malaria was killing patients.[6]

The WHO was reticent about artemisinin derivative use for several reasons: political (influence of the United States),[7] economic (increased cost), and scientific (medical research not corresponding to international standards). At the time, no pharmaceutical company was ready to invest in long, costly clinical trials, without hope of returns in the absence of official recommendations for use. At the end of 1993, the WHO organized its first informal consultation on "the role of artemisinin and its derivatives in malaria treatment." The recommendations were reminders that "artemisinin derivatives should only be prescribed in countries where poly-resistant *Plasmodium falciparum* was present; should not be commercialized in countries without poly-pharmacoresistance such as in Africa; should be administered in combination with another efficacious anti-malarial treatment; and should be followed up by a surveillance system to detect possible side effects, treatment efficacy, and maximize quality" (WHO, 1994: 1). The meeting targeted Asian countries, not Africa. The WHO stressed the shortcomings of scientific data on the inefficacy of standard treatments and avoided mentioning the political and economic pressures to which it was being subjected, particularly by the US government, which had little desire to leave the way open for a Chinese breakthrough.[8]

---

6 An estimated 80% to 90% of the million malaria deaths reported annually in the 1980s were among children in Africa.

7 MSF doctors, attending the International Tropical Medicine Conference (Thailand, 1992), recall American military doctors promoting MFQ and halofantrine at the same venue.

8 WHO director Gro Harlem Brundtland acknowledged these pressures in 2002, at a meeting with MSF senior staff and in the presence of WHO infectious diseases department directors, some of whom were American.

A second meeting was held in 1995 to "revise the group's recommendations and directives." The conclusions were limited to "the treatment of uncomplicated malaria and the use of antimalarials to protect travelers." While the WHO declared its concern about recent data showing reduced efficacy of standard treatments—particularly SP in Kenya, Tanzania, and Malawi—the use of artemisinin remained restricted to South East Asia: "At this time nothing justifies the use of oral or injectable forms of artemisinin in Africa as other efficacious treatments are available" (WHO, 1996, p. 57). The WHO also argued the need to avoid the "anarchistic" and "uncontrolled" arrival of artemisinin derivatives in Africa, citing the risk of a rapid decline in efficacy. In reality, artemisinin derivatives were already arriving in private pharmacies without any control of their usage, and they were being administered as monotherapies, favoring the rapid development of resistance.[9]

Quality documentation on malaria resistance in Africa was rare at the beginning of the 1990s. This was a direct consequence of low interest among scientific institutions, health ministries, and international organizations—including MSF. MSF and Epicentre had only conducted three resistance studies on the African continent from 1984 to 1997.[10] Some doctors had indeed observed resistances to treatment,[11] but found themselves out of their depth and without detailed knowledge about the state of scientific research at the time. Their worries were reinforced by particularly deadly epidemics in Kenya at the end of the 1990s.

---

9   The WHO only requested pharmaceutical companies to stop producing artemisinin derivate monotherapies a further ten years later, emphasising the role of governments in this domain. Of the twenty-three companies contacted, thirteen agreed to the request.

10   Moyo (Uganda) 1993, Tabou (Ivory Coast) 1995, and Benguela (Angola) in 1996.

11   In 1989, in Moyo, Uganda, the doctor and MSF–team leader wrote a report signalling malaria parasite resistance to chloroquine in the region, and the resulting difficulties in the treatment of uncomplicated malaria with available drugs.

Between January and May 1998, MSF intervened in response to a malaria epidemic that killed almost 4,000 people in the town of Wajir, Northeast Kenya (population 60,000). The epidemic probably caused 10,000 deaths in all at a district level (population 160,000) in association with malnutrition (Brown, 1998). At the same time, another epidemic started elsewhere in Kenya, in the Marsabit and Samburu districts. Standard malaria treatments were not brought into question, despite a Glaxo Wellcome study demonstrating a 60% treatment failure with chloroquine and complete efficacy for SP on the third day of treatment. It should be noted that the WHO recommends at least two weeks' follow-up to detect late treatment failures, and, as such, the study did not correspond to norms, and could not detect late failures (between four and fourteen days). That same year, Kenyan health authorities published a malaria treatment guide. It recommended SP as first-line treatment for uncomplicated malaria, except in areas where the parasite was still sensitive to chloroquine. Second-line treatment was either oral amodiaquine or oral quinine, and intravenous quinine was the reference for severe malaria.[12]

A worrying rise in the number of cases of malaria had been observed in the Kenyan high plateaus since 1990 (Mlakooti, 1998; Snow, 1999). MSF intervened late in the Kisii and Gucha districts (Nyanza province) from June to August 1999, after being asked for help by Merlin,[13] which was overwhelmed by the number of cases. The scale of the epidemic was such that the Kenyan army was called in to help medical relief in mid-July.

At the epidemic's peak, 600 patients were hospitalized at Kisii district hospital, 500 of whom were diagnosed with malaria. The hospital had a capacity of 250 beds, including 65 pediatric beds. Two hundred fifty of the 600 inpatients were children.

---

12   Ministry of Health, *National Guidelines for Diagnosis, Treatment and Prevention of Malaria for Health Workers*, Republic of Kenya, Nairobi, January 1998.

13   Merlin is an international medical NGO.

The number of blood transfusions increased from 80 to 340 per week. Similarly, at Ogembo hospital, which had 25 beds, 130 patients were hospitalized. At the same time, three mobile clinics treated 30,000 patients between July 19 and August 19 (Bracknell, 1999).

MSF developed its malaria epidemic response strategy during these interventions. First, MSF brought support to the two district hospitals (Kisii and Ogembo) and one health centre (Kembu Health Center), strengthening their inpatient capacities, recruiting personnel, performing training in severe malaria treatment, increasing transfusion capacities, and supplying anti-malarials, including notably artemether for severe cases. The Kenyan authorities had already accepted the use of artemether, and it was already present in hospitals and available to those who could pay for it. MSF realized that this level of intervention was not enough; action was needed earlier, before cases became severe and flooded hospitals and health centers. This led to the organization of mobile clinics, allowing rapid diagnosis and treatment for populations often living too far from health centers. This type of strategy corresponded to that used in the small epidemics on the Thai border, which aimed quickly to diagnose and treat a maximum number of cases in the hope of slowing or stopping transmission. The scale of the Kenyan epidemic meant that this hope was illusory— particularly so given that artemisinin derivatives were not being used as first-line treatment (one of the characteristics of artemisinin derivatives is to destroy sexual forms—gametocytes—of the parasite which are necessary for transmission of the disease by mosquitoes).

The Kenyan guide (1998) recommended changing to SP, but this had not occurred; information had been poorly transmitted and health personnel inadequately trained. Furthermore, there was a will to use up existing stocks of chloroquine in national pharmacies before the switch to SP, despite chloroquine resistance rates of up to 85%.

Artemisinin derivatives had not been completely forgotten, however. On the contrary, they were officially adopted by Kenyan health authorities on July 21, 1999, at a Malaria Task Force meeting presided by the director of Medical Services,[14] and this information was quickly transmitted to provincial authorities. The 1999 epidemic was nearing its end, and this decision may have been taken for political reasons, aiming to reduce the epidemic's political repercussions on central authorities. That said, at the end of July, for the last three weeks of the MSF's malaria intervention, a dose of artesunate was added to ambulatory SP treatment in mobile clinics. This led to the successful treatment of some patients, but was too late to affect the course of the epidemic.

The precedent for ACT use had been established. The Kenyan epidemic experience would become a reference point for strategies in the epidemics that followed: Burundi (2001), Sudan (2002), and Ethiopia (2004) (Checchi, 2006).

Bringing ACT to Africa

ACT was prescribed in MSF missions in Thailand beginning in 1994. The plan to use them in Africa was only formulated in 1999, however, and only started to become reality the following year. This time lag can be explained primarily by the obligation to respect national protocols. Any exceptions implied obtaining agreement from national health authorities. These decisions were difficult to influence in Africa, where there was much scientific uncertainty, and where ACT use had strong political and economic implications. The problem of drug supply also slowed the introduction of ACTs, very sparsely

---

14   The protocol associated AS and SP for one day.

available in Africa in the 1990s. Effort was required to ensure their production in sufficient quantities, their distribution, and to secure the corresponding national health ministry budget increases given their high relative cost compared to previous treatments. Scientifically, it could be comfortably argued that the continued use of monotherapies to which the parasite was significantly resistant would lead to a dead end in the short term (WHO, 2001). Chloroquine and SP treatment failure had not been clearly demonstrated by adequate studies, however, and immediate ACT use in Africa was controversial, even within MSF itself.[15] Finally, there were other, internal, reasons why MSF was unable to introduce ACTs, namely the need to prepare for the change through training and protocol changes.

Clinical Operational Research and Humanitarian Action

The pilot projects

From 1999 onwards, MSF aimed to introduce ACTs in all health centers where the association was operating, in collaboration with local health authorities. A number of steps needed to be taken: evaluation of the efficacy of existing treatments (data often lacking or impossible to interpret), material support (drug and diagnostic test supply), organization of prescriptive matters (diagnostic and therapeutic protocols, training), epidemiological data collection and analysis, and assessment of the new treatment in terms of efficacy and efficiency. These steps brought MSF practice into line with project follow-up and evaluation as required by evidence-based medicine, and reinforced MSF's arguments in discussions with ministries and international organizations, particularly the WHO.

An MSF doctor familiar with ACT use from his experience on the Thai border was given the role of lobbying for

15   From 2003, the international MSF movement was federated around the same strategy, and disagreements between operational sections were resolved through a malaria working group.

changes to national protocols. Right from the beginning it was a difficult process, particularly with the WHO. The institution is not, however, a monolith, and opinions differ according to departments. Although the Tropical Diseases Research program (TDR)[16] seemed to favor change, such was not the case at Roll Back Malaria (RBM).[17] Nevertheless, MSF began using artemisinin derivatives for the treatment of severe malaria in therapeutic feeding centers in Brazzaville, the Republic of Congo, in 2000. In 2001 MSF then introduced them for the treatment of uncomplicated malaria in Zambia, Liberia, and the Republic of Congo, followed by Sierra Leone, Burundi, and Kenya in 2002. There were difficulties though, as in October 2000, during a large-scale epidemic in the Burundian high plateaus, where MSF was quick to measure the failure of available treatment through resistance studies, hoping to convince national and international health authorities of the necessity of using ACTs. Unfortunately, MSF did not manage to convince either the Burundian authorities or the WHO.[18]

The opposition, skepticism, disorganization, and inertia often displayed by national and international authorities led MSF to increase the number of studies proving the inefficacy of national protocols in Africa. Studies to identify the best antimalarial to combine with ACTs were also organized between 2000 and 2004. They took place in pilot projects involving training in the use of rapid tests, data collection and analysis, and resistance studies comparing various ACT combinations.

Resistance studies

MSF and Epicentre launched a series of efficacy studies in collaboration with health ministries in the early 2000s to evaluate

16   Founded by the WHO in 1975.

17   The Roll Back Malaria network was created in 1998 as a WHO initiative in association with United Nations Children's Fund, the United Nations Development Programme, the World Bank, and other public and private partners.

18   See the chapter by M. Le Pape and I. Defourny in this book.

national protocols and support alternative propositions. A total of forty-three clinical studies in eighteen different countries were conducted by MSF and Epicentre between 2000 and 2004: eight in Asia and thirty-five in Africa, representing 25% of all field clinical studies conducted during this period (Guthmann, 2008 and 2009).

By setting up these efficacy studies, Epicentre and MSF highlighted WHO resistance-study protocols that in many circumstances underestimated treatment failure. MSF and Epicentre and the WHO and TDR subsequently worked together to improve assessment methodology (Guthmann et al., 2006).

In an orientation document for field teams (MSF, 2001) drawn up by an MSF doctor in charge of malaria, the arguments justifying ACT use in health centers supported by MSF in Africa were the following: the morbidity and mortality due to malaria; the emergence of resistance to the most commonly used antimalarials (chloroquine and SP) and subsequent treatment inefficacy; the potential public health effect of ACTs given their good results in treatment of the disease; the fight against resistance development and control of transmission.[19]

The introduction of rapid tests

In Thailand any suspicion of malaria was confirmed by biological examinations. In Africa, given the high number of cases and limited diagnostic means, treatment was often administered on clinical grounds. Laboratory confirmation is often impractical in isolated areas lacking staff and equipment, but it was the sheer number of malaria cases that often made laboratory testing difficult in health centers. The use of rapid tests needed to be validated, so Epicentre began a study in Mbarara, Uganda, in 2001. The objective was to compare various tests' performances in terms of sensitivity and

---

19 Artemisinin derivatives have a specific action against gametocytes. To transmit the disease, the anopheles mosquito feeds on infected blood containing gametocytes, which then evolve to an infectious form in its salivary glands and are injected at the next feed.

specificity, feasibility (ease of use in typical field conditions), and cost-efficacy. The rapid test in use at the time, specific for *Plasmodium falciparum*, was found to be very sensitive (96%), easy to use, and reasonably priced. It became MSF's standard.

Political Efforts

In the early 2000s, numerous studies were published showing the level of resistance to standard anti-malarial treatments in Africa. Furthermore, knowledge about the mechanisms and causes of resistance development increased, refuting the idea of continuing to treat malaria with single-drug therapies. This opened the way for MSF to intensify its plea in favor of ACTs. Health authorities nevertheless freely proposed combinations of older molecules (notably amodiaquine and SP)—"poor people's ACTs," as some described them—as a last effort against ACT introduction. MSF increased the number of scientific studies in response, which had the added advantage of obtaining initial authorizations to bring ACTs into different countries. MSF's insistence on ethical and scientific reasons (a doctor's duty to prescribe the best available treatment) forced economic and political issues to the background. MSF's inability to comprehend and master these factors severely hampered progress on the issue of ACT.

Plasmodium falciparum malaria cases increased markedly in KwaZulu-Natal province, South Africa, between 1995 and 2000, linked with development of resistance to insecticides and to SP (which had replaced chloroquine in 1998). In 2001, a year after the reintroduction of DDT spraying of houses, large-scale insecticide-impregnated mosquito net distribution, and the introduction of ACTs, hospitalizations and deaths due to malaria dropped by 89%. Malaria incidence also dropped by 85% in sentinel sites. These reductions were confirmed in the years that followed. The presentation of these results at an internal MSF conference in October 2002 (Barnes et al., 2005) had a considerable effect in removing resistance to ACT use within the association. The meeting report concluded "we have a tendency to concentrate on external obstacles, but there is also significant resistance to the use of ACTs within the association" (MSF, 2002).

During the Third Multilateral Initiative on Malaria–Pan African Malaria Conference in Arusha, Tanzania, in November 2002, a debate was held on the subject "How can expensive but essential drugs be made accessible to those in need ?" The Zambian health ministry representative asked the assembly if the question was whether an African child's life was worth 2.4 dollars.[20] Because the time for cheap (i.e., ineffective) drugs for poor people was a thing of the past, what were we waiting for to make effective treatments accessible in Africa? "The World Bank is here, at this table, and seems to be saying that the money is there!" Furthermore, several attendees were surprised that multinational drug companies had discouraged artesunate production in Tanzania, where the *Artemisia* plantations growing not far from Arusha were of high quality, and contained more artemisinin than Chinese productions. The crop was being exported to the USA (where they were trying to synthesize the drug) and Europe. Naturally, the cost of the drug would have been much lower if produced in Tanzania.

In 2002, several East African states thought about changing national malaria treatment protocols and introducing transition strategies. The choices generally were not made based on efficacy, but on financial criteria, negotiated between governments and donors. MSF and the Campaign for Access to Essential Medicines wrote a report on the costs of ACT introduction.

---

20   The lowest-priced ACT at the time was $1.50, whereas chloroquine or SP cost around $0.10.

According to the report, "it is governments' responsibility to modify malaria treatment protocols so as to offer efficacious treatment to patients in need. If we examine existing national health budgets and available international aid, it is financially possible to rapidly introduce ACTs where medically indicated" (Kindermans, 2002).

The report was a reference point at a press conference held in Nairobi on February 13, 2002. The idea was to show the real costs of ACT-based protocols and thereby motivate national program directors and international donors to adopt the approach. The additional cost of ACT introduction for the five East African countries with the highest levels of resistance (Burundi, Kenya, Rwanda, Tanzania, and Uganda) was estimated at $19 million a year. According to MSF representatives, this was not insurmountable once donors recognized the importance of introducing efficacious combinations. The need to expand the ACT market to reduce the cost of the drugs was also stressed.

At the same time, American researchers were attempting chemically to synthesize artemisinin, aiming to increase production independently of the constraints of wormwood cultivation. The economic return was to be reaped through patent applications.

The situation changed when the Global Fund to Fight AIDS, Tuberculosis and Malaria[21] declared in 2004 that it would only finance projects using ACTs from that point onwards. The WHO followed in 2006 with a new guide on malaria treatment. New funds appeared from donor countries keen to protect themselves against the potential menace, ending a scientific debate that had become obsolete. Public health institutions' access to a new and essential effective treatment does not automatically mean ACT administration to patients at high risk of death, however.

21 The Global Fund was created in 2002.

Several Epicentre and MSF studies have shown that despite the introduction of ACTs into national protocols, patients still had little access to them. Aware of the limits, MSF worked on simplifying the prescription and reducing the costs of ACT through the Drugs for Neglected Diseases Initiative. Working in collaboration with Sanofi-Aventis, a combination (ASAQ) was commercialized in 2007: for the first time a child could be treated with a single tablet once a day[22] for three days for less than half a dollar.

Even when recommended by the WHO and integrated into national treatment protocols, effective treatments, once in national central stocks, are not readily available to small children. Public health strategies are needed to produce consensus, transmit national recommendations to all levels of health systems, and ensure continual long-lasting implementation. Should a medical humanitarian organization such as MSF engage in the processes of negotiations, persuasion, standardization, and economic planning? Are such procedures not outside the organization's scope? Success in persuasion means having knowledge of local structures and traditions, along with social and political willpower, and the ability to galvanize national institutions. To make treatments accessible to those most in need—those who do not necessarily seek help from healthcare structures—pressure must continue to be placed on international donors and the pharmaceutical industry.

---

22 The tablet's dosage form permits easy dissolution in water and administration with a spoon, often indispensible for correct ingestion by small children.

Bibliography

Balkan, S. 2003. *MSF: ACT Implementation proposal.* Paris: Médecins Sans Frontières.

Barnes, K. I., D.N. Durrheim, F. Little, A. Jackson, U. Mehta, E. Allen, S.S. Dlamini, J. Tsoka, B. Bredenkamp, D.J. Mthembu, N.J. White, B.L Sharp. 2005. "Effect of Artemether-Lumefantrine Policy and Improved Vector Control on Malaria Burden in KwaZulu–Natal, South Africa." *Plos Medicine* 2 (11) e330: 1123–1134.

Bracknell, S. 1999. *Emergency intervention for Curative assistance and Epidemic control of a Malaria outbreak in Kisii and Gucha disctricts, Nyanza province, Kenya, June 20–August 20 1999.* Internal report. Médecins Sans Frontières.

Brown, V., M. A. Issak, M. Rossi, P. Barboza, A. Paugam. 1998. "Epidemic of malaria in north-eastern Kenya." *The Lancet* 352 (9137): 1356–1357.

Checchi, F., J. Cox, S. Balkan, A. Tamrat, G. Priotto, K. Alberti, D. Zurovac, J.-P. Guthmann. 2006. "Malaria Epidemics and Interventions, Kenya, Burundi, Southern Sudan, and Ethiopia, 1999–2004." *Emerging Infectious Diseases* 12 (10): 1477–1485.

Fogg, C., 2001. *Malaria in Kisii and Gucha districts, Nyanza province, Western Kenya. Surveillance and prevalence studies in preparation for malaria outbreak.* Paris: Epicentre.

Fogg, C., F. Bajunirwe, P. Piola, S. Biraro, F. Checchi, J. Kiguli, P. Namiro, J. Musabe, A. Kyomugisha, J-P Guthman. 2004. "Adherence to a six-dose regimen of arthemether-lumefantrine for treatment of. uncomplicated *Plasmodium Falciparum* malaria in Uganda." *The American Journal of Tropical Medicine and Hygiene* 71 (5): 525–30.

Gerstl, S., S. Cohuet, F. Checchi, 2004. *Traitement du paludisme par une combinaison d'artésunate et d'amodiaquine-Evaluation de son utilisation par la population. Province de Makamba, Burundi.* Médecins Sans Frontières and Epicentre in collaboration with the Ministry of Public Health of Burundi.

Guthmann, J.-P., L. Pinoges, F. Checchi, S. Cousens, S. Balkan, M. Van Herp, D. Legros, P. Olliaro. 2006. "Methodological issues in the assessment of antimalarial drug treatment: analysis of 13 studies in eight African countries from 2001 to 2004." *Antimicrobial Agents and Chemotherapy* 50 (11): 3734–3739.

Guthmann, J.-P., F. Checchi, I Van den Broek, S. Balkan, M. Van Herp, E. Comte, O. Bernal, J-M Kindermans, S. Venis, D. Legros, P. Guerin. 2008. "Assessing Antimalarial Efficacy in a time of Change to Artemisinine-based Combination Therapies: The Role of Médecins Sans Frontières." *Plos Medicine* 5 (8): 1191–1199.

Guthmann, J.-P. 2009. "Recherche clinique et action humanitaire. Le rôle de Médecins Sans Frontières dans la lutte contre le paludisme." *Médecine/Science* 25 (3): 301–306.

Hook, C., 2007. *A job half done? Implementation of the MSF policy on falciparum malaria 2002–2006*, Internal Report for Médecins Sans Frontières Operations and Medical Departments. Geneva.

Kindermans, J.-M. 2002. *Nouveaux protocoles nationaux pour le traitement du paludisme en Afrique: à quel coût et qui paiera ? Études de cas: Burundi, Kenya, Rwanda, Tanzanie et Ouganda.* Campaign for Access to Essential Medicines, Médecins Sans Frontières.

Luxemburger, C., F. O. Ter Kuile, F. Nosten, G. Dolan, J.-H. Bradol, L. Phaipun, T.Chongsuphajaisiddhi, N. J. White. 1994. "Single day mefloquine-artesunate combination in the treatment of multi-drug resistant falciparum malaria." *Transactions of the Royal Society of Tropical Medicine and Hygiene* 88 (2): 213–217.

Mlakooti, M. A., K. Biomndo, G.D. Shanks. 1998. "Reemergence of epidemic malaria in the Highlands of Western Kenya." *Emerging Infectious Diseases* 4 (4): 671–676.

Médecins Sans Frontières (MSF). 2001. *Treatment of non-complicated Plasmodium falciparum malaria in MSF missions in Africa.* Medical department (Suna Balkan), Paris, October 24.

——. 2002. *Malaria workshop, final report*, Brussels.

——. 2008. *Améliorer l'accès aux traitements efficaces contre le palu-*

disme au Mali. Expérience positive de réduction de la barrière financière pour les patients dans le cercle de Kangaba. Bruxelles: Médecins Sans Frontières OCB.

Nosten, F., M. Van Vugt, R. Price, C. Luxemburger, K.L. Thway, A. Brockman, R. McGready, F. Ter Kuile, S. Looareesuwan, N.J. White. 2000. "Effects of artesunate-mefloquine combination on incidence of *Plasmodium falciparum* malaria and mefloquine resistance in western Thailand: a prospective study." *The Lancet* 356 (9226): 297–302.

Piola, P., C. Fogg, F. Bajunirwe, S. Biraro, F. Grandesso, E. Ruzagira, J. Babigumira, I. Kigozi, J. Kiguli, J. Kyomuhendo, L. Ferradini, W. Taylor, F. Checchi, J.P. Guthmann. 2005. "Supervised versus unsupervised intake of six-dose artemether-lumefantrine for treatment of acute, uncomplicated *Plasmodium falciparum* malaria in Mbarara, Uganda: a randomised trial." *The Lancet* 365 (9469): 1467–1473.

Prescrire. 2007. "Traitements à base d'artémisinine en Afrique. Lenteurs, progrès et lacunes." *La Revue Prescrire* 290: 939–940.

Snow, R. W., A. Ikoku, J. Omumbo, J. Ouma. 1999. *The epidemiology, politics and control of malaria epidemics in Kenya: 1900–1998.* Roll Back Malaria, World Health Organization.

Snow, R. W. 2004. "Malaria the invisible victims." *Nature* 430: 934–935.

World Health Organization (WHO). 1994. *Antimalarial drug policies: data requirements, treatment of uncomplicated malaria and the management of malaria in pregnancy*, WHO/MAL/94.1070. Geneva.

——. 1996. *Prise en charge du paludisme non compliqué. Rapport d'une consultation informelle, Genève, 18-21 septembre 1995*, WHO/MAL/96.1075.

——. 2001. *Les combinaisons thérapeutiques antipaludiques. Rapport d'une consultation technique de l'OMS*, WHO/CDS/RBM/2001.35.

——. 2008. *World Malaria Report.* Geneva: World Health Organization.

Chapter 9

AIDS

A New Pandemic Leading to
New Medical and Political Practices

Jean-Hervé Bradol and Elizabeth Szumilin

By the late 1990s the mortality rate for the human immuno-deficiency virus (HIV) had been brought under control in high-income countries, thanks to the combination of several antiretroviral drugs. Yet there was no plan for administering the treatment in the world's largest foci of infection. Sub-Saharan Africa in particular, the most seriously affected region, was not benefiting from therapeutic advances. Refusing to accept this situation required innovative efforts on two fronts: medical and political. In 2008, 140,000 people, ten thousand of them children, received free generic antiretroviral drugs in projects supported by MSF. After a limited number of laboratory tests, patients are prescribed fixed-dose combination treatments (in a single tablet) by non-specialist doctors or nurses. If there are no complications, the prescriptions can sometimes be renewed by public health technicians.[1] Treatment of opportunistic infections is available wherever possible, and treatment for tuberculosis, the leading cause of death among AIDS patients in Africa, is integrated with HIV treatment. During the first few years of treatment, survival rates are similar to those obtained in North America and Western Europe. Does this qualify as a success? Only a sustained reduction in the number of deaths and the number of

---

[1] As compared with France, where fewer than ninety thousand people receive *Affection de longue durée* (long-term illness) health insurance for AIDS and only specialist physicians can prescribe antiretroviral therapy.
See www.sante-sports.gouv.fr/IMG//pdf/03_Epidemiologie.pdf (in French).

people carrying the virus in the hardest-hit regions will show the true effect of the changes that have occurred in recent years. This article presents the circumstances and reasons which led MSF to treat patients who would not otherwise have access to new and costly treatments.

The Right Circumstances, and a Certain Indifference

According to the World Health Organization (WHO), "The human immunodeficiency virus (HIV) is a retrovirus that infects cells of the human immune system, destroying or impairing their function. In the early stages of infection, the person has no symptoms. However, as the infection progresses, the immune system becomes weaker, and the person becomes more susceptible to opportunistic infections. The most advanced stage of HIV infection is acquired immunodeficiency syndrome (AIDS). It can take ten to fifteen years for an HIV-infected person to develop AIDS. Antiretroviral drugs can slow down the process even further. HIV is transmitted through unprotected sexual intercourse (anal or vaginal), transfusion of contaminated blood, sharing of contaminated needles, and between a mother and her infant during pregnancy, childbirth, and breastfeeding."[2]

A look at the advance in knowledge on HIV from the early 1980s to the mid-1990s shows that discoveries were made quickly (Grmek, 1990). Clinicians began to suspect the existence of a new disease in 1981. In 1982, transmission of the disease to hemophiliacs via blood products that, despite filtering, transmitted the infectious agent suggested a very small micro-organism: a virus. In 1983, HIV was classified as a member of the retrovirus family because of its mode of replication. It was cloned in 1984, and its genome was identified. The identification of HIV antigens led to a blood test that—within certain limits of sensi-

2   http://www.who.int/topics/hiv_aids/en/index.html.

tivity and specificity—could confirm or rule out the presence of HIV (1985), making it possible to prevent transmission through blood transfusions. The test identified those who carried the virus and those who did not. It then became possible to discern better how the virus spread within populations, and to identify the most seriously affected regions and the highest risk groups and behaviors. This helped define and measure the effect of the preventive actions that were being introduced in high-income countries in the late 1980s. Understanding the retroviral mode of replication led to the use of the first drug, Zidovudine, whose efficacy is relative and temporary (1987). Prevention of mother-to-child HIV transmission and administration of a treatment against the virus itself became possible. Knowing HIV's genetic makeup also led to measurement of the viral load in the blood—a key laboratory indicator for monitoring treatment efficacy. Genetics also enabled identification of mutant viruses resistant to certain drugs, making it possible to avoid ineffective antiretrovirals right from the start of treatment. Understanding the virus' predilection for certain blood cells involved in the immune response resulted in a test that could measure HIV's effect on the body's immune defenses, the T4 lymphocyte level (CD4 test). At the same time, different strains of the virus (HIV-1, HIV-2, etc.) were identified. Roughly fifteen years separated the first clinical diagnoses (1981) from the prescription of a treatment transforming an almost-always fatal disease into a chronic one (1996).

The 1983 International AIDS Conference in Denver saw the emergence of a political movement for people living with HIV. At the 1989 Montreal Conference, ACT UP and its Canadian counterpart, AIDS Action Now, manifested their presence as soon as the opening ceremony started. They demanded that research focus on patients' needs rather than on pharmaceutical industry interests alone. In 1994 the principle that organizations of people living with HIV should have greater participation in the fight against AIDS was adopted by forty-two countries at a summit in Paris. In 2008 the Global Network of People living with HIV (GNP+) included more than a thousand member organizations. They demand participation in all institutional processes regarding the fight against AIDS, call for universal access to prevention and treatment programs, and emphasize prevention targeting those who are HIV-positive. They also call for more information on sexual and reproductive health, are opposed to criminalization of virus transmission, and defend the rights of people living with HIV.

In 1989 MSF-France's Board of Directors approved a proposal to participate in the Montreal AIDS Conference, and MSF-Belgium opened a free, anonymous testing center in Brussels. The MSF delegate to the Montreal Conference declared that it was "unthinkable to him that Médecins Sans Frontières should not be involved in the response to AIDS." He suggested possible approaches involving education, treatment, epidemiological surveys, and palliative care. He reported that treatments were being developed "based on very complex and very expensive combinations" and, among the avenues of research, he noted that there were "openings in Africa on mother-to-child transmission. ... A long debate began between those who thought that Médecins Sans Frontières could and should conduct AIDS-related activities, and those who thought it was not within the organization's scope."[3] The debate was lively and tense. Advocates of engagement emphasized the large number of deaths in certain social categories and certain areas of the world—Africa in particular. They spoke of possible prevention activities and treatment approaches. Those resistant to the proposal stressed that there were no drugs available, and that prevention activities relying primarily on persuading people to change their sexual behavior had very doubtful outcomes. In their view, MSF—a

3   Report from the MSF-France Board of Directors meeting, June 30, 1989.

foreign organization with little mastery of the languages needed for disseminating information and a superficial approach to local culture—was not the institution best-suited to do work that was more social than medical. The first report on AIDS, written by Epicentre[4] for MSF in 1990, concerned the situation in France: "MSF is frequently asked to intervene on AIDS in France. Yet no one in the organization is particularly responsible or expert in that area, and MSF has no policy on the subject."[5] The requests were coming from patient organizations, researchers, and practitioners hoping that MSF would support their cause with its resources and reputation. A large diversity of opinions emerged among the governing bodies at MSF. Over the 1980s, these bodies had developed into a movement of different national sections (Belgium, Spain, Greece, Switzerland, Holland, etc.). The relative political indifference at the office in Paris was met with internal opposition that had a lot of support from other national sections.

In missions outside France, the growing awareness of how health care facilities were responsible for the spread of AIDS led to a series of measures aimed at preventing virus transmission during medical procedures. In June 1993 the medical department at the Paris headquarters informed the Board of Directors that screening tests were being set up at sites where MSF was directly responsible for transfusions. While members of the Board are not directly in charge of sensitive activities (sterilizations, transfusions, injections, surgery, etc.), this work is nevertheless dependent on them. An unanticipated diagnosis before transfusion, coupled with the fear of stigmatization and discrimination and no offer of treatment, has sometimes meant that testing was delayed. Studies of serological prevalence among pregnant women (Uganda and Sudan) sparked a debate on the appropriateness of informing a woman that she is HIV-positive

---

4   Epicentre is an MSF satellite organization that specializes in the epidemiology of intervention, research, and training.

5   Philippe Malfait, *Mission MSF et sida en France*, Epicentre, January 25, 1990.

during a routine pre-natal consultation. "What should we do with someone whom we've informed, after our testing, that she is HIV-positive, or with a patient? We risk condemning people to a faster and more painful death, because that knowledge will get them ostracized from their community."[6]

Antiretroviral drugs made their first appearance in an MSF HIV prevention kit in the mid-1990s, following an accidental occupational exposure to blood. Mutual aid was also discreetly provided to infected colleagues, friends, and lovers. MSF employees with opportunistic infections were given access on an individual basis to treatments that were unavailable, and often very expensive, in their own countries. Ad hoc networks sprang up to stay with dying friends and loved ones. Refusals to grant visas on the grounds of seropositivity were circumvented with the organization's complicity. Later, when the first triple therapies appeared, they were sent "under the counter" to colleagues in countries where they were unavailable. Such actions were limited in number, but they highlighted the fact that MSF needed to get involved in treating the disease. One of the very first field projects (Surin, Thailand, 1995) that focused on treatment, rather than prevention, was started by an expatriate nurse who had spent several years supporting Thai friends in the terminal stage of the disease. From such individual acts, carried out in the belief that therapeutic solidarity was morally legitimate, emerged a sense of political affinity among those who strongly opposed an institutional position they considered overly timid, and who were willing to change MSF's policy. Some members of MSF hoped for public advocacy and the large-scale use of antiretroviral drugs as a way to reconcile individual experience and institutional action.

The epidemic was particularly severe in places (eastern, southern, and central Africa) where MSF had developed its original, non-AIDS-related hospital activities. The medical teams

6   Report from the June 1989 Board of Directors meeting, Paris.

were faced with a growing number of cases involving difficult-to-treat opportunistic infections and management-intensive terminal patients. The teams also had to deal with local staff who were not informed of how the virus was transmitted, and who refused to care for patients for fear of infection. MSF team members mobilized to improve patient welcome and disseminate basic knowledge on transmission and prevention with information and professional training sessions. Practical objectives included welcoming patients, treating opportunistic infections, and providing palliative care (pain, wounds, nutritional support, personal hygiene, psychological and social support). Antiretroviral drugs are therefore essential. Without them, treatment is difficult and ill adapted, and neither reduces the body's viral load nor restores the immune system. This was an argument for their use.

Prevention activities in the field increased among specific groups, such as prostitutes and truck drivers in Mwanza, Malawi, despite the reluctance of some, who wanted to focus mainly on treatment. In late 1995 an editorial on the cover of MSF France's in-house magazine *Messages* asked, "MSF: a white, heterosexual, HIV-negative organization?" It was a provocative title designed to promote prevention activities and patient support, and fight against stigmatization and discrimination. Such activities were not widely adopted by MSF-France, but began to flourish among other sections. By 1998 MSF was able to claim "48 field projects in which AIDS is a major component." Without an effective treatment, however, the fight against discrimination and in favor of prevention was not enough to make AIDS a core concern in MSF's policy.

Drug Prescription: Hesitations and Audacity

At the opening ceremony of the 1996 International AIDS Conference in Vancouver, the New York representative for ACT UP raised the issue of access to treatment for the hardest-hit populations. "Yes, the preliminary results from these hugely expensive combination treatments look great. But we are a long way from a cure, even for the rich who can afford the treatments. And we are no closer to a cure for the majority of people living with AIDS on this planet than we were ten years ago. Most peoples living with AIDS can't get aspirins." [7]

At the 1997 Abidjan Conference, the French president and the minister of health called for "international therapeutic solidarity." In June 1997, with support from a few multinational drug companies and the World Bank, the Joint United Nations Programme on HIV/AIDS (UNAIDS, created in 1995) launched the *HIV Drug Access Initiative* (UNAIDS-DAI). The DAI relied on some of the big pharmaceutical firms agreeing to differential pricing according to a country's income level, whereas these firms previously asked a single price worldwide. In 1998 several countries (Uganda, Senegal, and Ivory Coast) began using triple therapy in their public programs. Its virological efficacy was established in the initial reports. These early experiences using triple therapies in resource-limited countries proved their feasibility and efficacy. Some of the practical aspects (the lack of generics; prices that were still too high; asking patients to contribute to the cost; the lack of fixed-dose combination of three antiretroviral drugs in a single pill; the significant clinical, laboratory, and psychosocial follow-up needed; etc.) were only compatible with cohorts of several hundred patients, however, at a time when tens of thousands of patients were waiting for the simplest, least expensive treatment.

The small number of patients treated by the UNAIDS accelerated-access initiative contrasted with the experience in Brazil, whose national program—using generics and free medications—rapidly treated nearly 100,000 patients (170,000 in 2008). In 1996 Brazil launched a public treatment program by presidential

---

7   http://www.actupny.org/Vancouver/sawyerspeech.html.

decree. Brazilian patent law allows for compulsory licensing (without the patent-holder's consent) to produce generic drugs, so while the public pharmaceutical company Pharmanguinhos (Oswaldo Cruz Foundation) does not manufacture all antiretrovirals itself, the possibility of doing so—should a private firm's price be considered too high—creates a credible threat of competition that lowers prices. Brazil stands out because it was the first low- or medium-income country to treat large numbers of patients, and remained the only one to do so until the mid-2000s. MSF reached an agreement with Brazil's public institutions to export Brazilian antiretrovirals to South Africa. Apart from this agreement, Brazil has never supported the effort to treat patients in very poor countries by exporting generics,[8] though it does assist them in developing their own production.

The high cost of the triple therapies used by Brazil (about $3,000 per patient per year) made large-scale initiatives by other countries highly unlikely. In February 2000 the Indian pharmaceutical company Cipla[9] announced that it would be marketing a combination treatment, Triomune, for $350 per patient per year. Its components were chosen based on efficacy, the amount of time until certain side effects appeared, and, above all, the price of raw materials.[10] The aim at the time was to offer it at the lowest possible price: $650 per patient per year, as opposed to several thousand dollars. Cipla granted MSF an additional $300 discount, which was ultimately extended to all customers. It was not in the economic interest of the patent-holders of each individual drug to manufacture a single pill, so producing generics without a patent made it possible to produce the triple therapy.

8   The World Trade Organization (WTO) has allowed countries to manufacture generic drugs legally for public health reasons, but the possibility of sending these generic drugs to other countries where they are covered by patents is unclear.

9   Cipla's creation in 1935 expressed the nationalism of its founder, Khwaja Abdul Hamied. The company was honored by a visit by Mahatma Gandhi in 1939.

10   Telephone interview with Dr. Yusuf Hamied, Cipla chairman and CEO, January 23, 2009.

This was the first time patients throughout the world had access to such a simple treatment—three antiretroviral drugs in a single tablet, morning and evening. Triomune's low price and ease of use opened the way for public health programs on a national scale.

At the same time, in Africa, private companies from various sectors (mining, energy, beverage, automotive, etc.) began funding access to antiretroviral drugs for their employees. Held in one of the most seriously affected countries, the July 2000 International AIDS Conference in Durban was a high point in improving access to treatment. It was at this venue that Merck, the pharmaceutical giant, and the Bill and Melinda Gates Foundation announced their $100 million donation for a treatment program in Botswana. The hype surrounding these philanthropic actions masked the essential fact that even the least expensive triple therapies, available through UNAIDS, were nevertheless still very costly (between $800 and $1,000). Information obtained from the pharmaceutical industry, and confirmed by a WHO expert, prompted MSF to publish the report *HIV/AIDS Medicines Pricing* (Perez-Casas, 2000), which showed that it would be possible to reduce the cost to under $200 per patient per year.

Procuring the drugs and getting them to the field meant clearing a dual pharmaceutical and legal hurdle (Boulet, 1999). No internationally recognized reference institution could guarantee the quality of the supply source alternatives to the pharmaceutical multinationals. Buyers were unlikely to be reassured by generic triple therapies from India, which were not marketed in either the US or Europe. MSF criticized the WHO for not taking responsibility; humanitarian pharmacists had to visit and validate manufacturing sites themselves in order to choose suppliers. In 2001 MSF began publishing an international guide to purchasing antiretroviral drugs for developing countries (the Campaign for Access to Essential Medicines, MSF, 2008). MSF-Logistique's legal status as a pharmaceutical establishment facilitated transit through Europe and redistribution in several dozen countries. To manage the risks involved in purchasing, storing, importing, and exporting generic triple therapies, MSF recruited a team of lawyers and pharmacists specialized in intellectual property issues, administrative registration, supplier selection, and drug marketing.

Just because a treatment is available on the market does not mean that authorities will automatically approve—or medical teams support—its use. Obtaining official authorization and convincing medical teams of the benefits means that new products need to be incorporated into a treatment protocol that is realistic both in terms of the patients' circumstances and the caregivers' professional practice. How to simplify without sacrificing efficacy? That was the task of the staff at MSF's medical departments, charged with providing technical support for field teams, with backup from experts at university medical centers. Some of the doctors who undertook this technical adaptation had continued to take short-term assignments in hospitals in Europe, Japan, Australia, or North America, and had been prescribing triple therapy for several years. With their experiences in resource-limited countries in mind, they were convinced that the protocols could be simplified without sacrificing the practices essential to therapeutic efficacy. Brazil had already proven that it was possible to prescribe antiretroviral drugs in middle-income countries, and others were following the same path, particularly Thailand. There were strong reservations, however, about sub-Saharan Africa, which, over the past decades, had suffered increasing poverty, political instability, and the collapse of public health institutions.

There were some parameters the medical team could control, such as prescription quality and drug management, but if patients didn't take medication regularly, failure was inevitable. From an individual stand point, patients facing imminent death would have more to gain by trying a treatment that is risky; but a poorly controlled program and bad treatment compliance (creating resistant strains of the virus) would compromise the future of treatment for the population as a whole. For this reason, the patient's ability to come for check-ups (distance, available transportation, and budget) was an essential criterion for acceptance into the group receiving triple therapy. A strict treatment protocol means more than just coming in for check-ups, however. The patient must also understand, or at least accept, the medical reasons underlying the protocol. The MSF medical team decided to focus on providing information to the patients using specialized medical counselors, and a member of the patient's social circle was chosen and trained to encourage daily adherence to treatment.

Lab testing was also a tricky issue. Existing knowledge suggested starting antiretroviral drugs when the immune response was markedly weakened, but lab tests were not readily accessible to MSF teams. Other tests to evaluate the function of potential target organs for side effects were also needed. Monitoring treatment efficacy would have required lab tests to measure viral replication in the body (the number of viruses per unit of blood, or viral load). In a professional setting dominated by the idea of evidence-based medicine which often relies on the measurement of biological markers, initiating treatment based on a marked deterioration in immune defenses, ensuring its efficacy, and preventing its toxicity without the help of lab tests seemed dangerously experimental.

Once the protocols were defined and administrative authorization obtained, there were still several concerns hindering prescription. Would the fact that there were only a small number of treatments available for a large number of patients lead to tensions, violence, or crime? Should priority be given to people who were needed to treat others (doctors, nurses, etc.), or even to those who performed essential societal functions (political leaders, teachers, etc.)? Decisions to launch field projects were based on several criteria: the local prevalence of AIDS, the attitude of public health officials (whether they were open to the use of antiretroviral drugs), and MSF's institutional interests. Treatments were administered to patients who were already frequenting outpatient clinics and hospital services, with priority going to those whose condition was most critical. Medical staff would be among the first to receive treatment due to their proximity with those prescribing it. Tensions did exist, and MSF sometimes hesitated to treat its own staff. The impossibility of delegating the treatment of MSF personnel to specialized institutions, which were largely non-existent, was a convincing argument. Being able to prescribe such complicated-to-manage treatments simultaneously in the dozens of countries where MSF intervened was difficult. Some in MSF's leadership feared that adopting an official resolution in favor of treating staff when there was no treatment mechanism in place might expose the organization to legal action by employees. Finally, in November 2002, the MSF International Council decided to guarantee MSF employees access to antiretroviral treatment.

Political Dynamics

By the early 1990s infectious diseases had again become a priority in international relations due to their potential economic and security repercussions. The emergence of new epidemics (Ebola and AIDS, in particular) and the fear of bioterrorism spurred governments to step up their disease-related activities. Many institutions (national governments, international organizations, pharmaceutical firms, national and international private organizations, religious institutions, unions, political parties, etc.) were faced with the dilemma of how to respond to the AIDS pandemic. The Internet played a key role in relationships that transcended borders, spreading to the most peripheral players (patients, caregivers, citizens), and reaching the top of public health, economic, and political institutions. Until then, the issues of drug access had been examined behind closed doors, and were the exclusive domain of experts, manufacturers, and government representatives. Henceforth, the discussion enjoyed broad media exposure. AIDS organizations and medical organizations like MSF took their place at the negotiating table. The medical and political dynamics challenged interpretation according to institutional positions or individual opinions based on their own interests. The strong feelings around the disease changed the usual dividing lines between individuals and institutions. We can define three basic attitudes: realism, universalism, and caution.

The realists argued that the conditions necessary for increasing the number of people treated from a few hundred thousand to several million did not exist. Drug availability by itself could not make up for the patients' lack of schooling, the shortage of qualified personnel and equipment, the meager budgets and inadequate management of health care institutions, or the poverty and instability of the hardest-hit countries. Why make a special effort for AIDS and not for other diseases that were just as prevalent, even more deadly, and far easier to treat? MSF, an emergency-oriented organization, would not have the expertise and constancy that were essential for a lifetime commitment to the patient. There was a serious risk that drugs would be used incorrectly and that mutant, antiretroviral-resistant strains of the virus would rapidly emerge. Prescribing before conditions were right would compromise the ability to introduce treatment under more favorable circumstances in the future. Another perverse effect—a drop in prices, and, more importantly, a weakening of intellectual property rights—would discourage research and development funding for new drugs.

The prospect of a return on investment would be undermined by black market imports of low-price generics competing with patented drugs in viable markets, and by an erosion of profit margins in emerging markets due to lower, differential pricing based on country income. Charitable donation was proposed as the only suitable method in the rare situations where conditions were right for using triple therapy. At the 2000 International AIDS Conference in Durban, Merck announced that it would supply two antiretroviral drugs free of charge for the national treatment program in Botswana. In that country, where one in four adults (fifteen to fifty years old) carried the virus, realism, faced with a potential demographic catastrophe, met its limits.

Universalists advocated making AIDS treatment accessible to everyone. Public health policies could not be restricted to priority groups dictated by disease statistics. Indeed, societies' reactions to the pandemic, whether rational or not, would be an opportunity for poorly functioning health care systems to use the fight against AIDS as a starting point for recovery. Generally speaking, the universalists characterized any objection to making HIV treatment immediately accessible as an obstacle to be overcome. The MSF representative who participated in the parallel meetings at the 1999 WTO Ministerial Conference in Seattle declared that patients were dying not from AIDS, but from the unavailability of drugs due to the patent system. This reasoning, without limiting it to the realm of intellectual property alone, supposes a change in attitude by governments, the pharmaceutical industry, the medical profession, and patients.

Where the universalists saw obstacles to overcome, the cautious needed guarantees before taking action. Precautions had to be taken in order to satisfy not only the moral imperative to treat, but also the need to do no harm, and to avoid squandering available resources and compromising the future. So prescribing HIV treatment was considered, but on a smaller scale and in countries that already had some means (Brazil and Thailand, for example) and depending on the environment (patents, the policy of patient contribution, limited human and material resources, etc.). The first use of antiretroviral drugs in Africa on the initiative of UNAIDS, and the first MSF protocols, illustrate this cautious approach.

All three attitudes brought morality, medical science, public health, economic rationalism, and political will to bear in their arguments; all three wanted to be universal, realistic, and cautious at the same time. In practice, however, they were mutually contradictory. Compromise was essential, but finding the perfect balance was impossible. MSF was a good example of this dynamic plurality of opinions that changed as a function of many variables, some more heavily weighted than others: the emergence of triple therapy, the will of governments, social and political mobilization, the changing application of intellectual property rules, the drop in antiretroviral prices, the availability of public funding, the analysis of the early experiences in the field, scientific publications, public controversies, and each institution's own interests.

Governments, international organizations, pharmaceutical firms, and local associations were all involved in a national and international political dynamic that exposed their contradictions, obliged them to explain themselves publicly, and forced them to make decisions that, until previously, they had considered contrary to their intentions and their interests. In May 2000 President Clinton supported the countries of sub-Saharan Africa that wished to produce and import generic drugs (Executive Order 13155). In July 2000 at the United Nations (UN) Security Council meeting and the Group of Eight (G8) summit in Okinawa, two important commitments were made: "mobilizing additional resources" and "addressing the complex issue of access to medicines in developing countries, and assessing obstacles being faced by developing countries."[11] The terms "access" and "obstacles" in the final G8 resolution were borrowed from the vocabulary of non-governmental organizations, including MSF, that were involved in preparing the Okinawa summit. Then UN Security Council Resolution 1308 (2000) stressed that "the HIV/AIDS pandemic, if unchecked, may pose a risk to stability and security." The World Bank described AIDS as a "development crisis."

After the failure of the WTO Ministerial Conference in Seattle (1999) there was strong pressure to ensure that the Doha Conference (2001) provide a solution to the crisis. The question of access to drugs seemed to offer the possibility of a positive outcome for at least one of the issues being negotiated internationally. The monopoly granted to patent holders for marketing their drugs was weighing heavily on prices; in the late 1990s, triple therapy cost between $10,000 and $15,000 a year. Therefore, what was needed was to make application of the Trade-related Aspects of Intellectual Property Rights (TRIPS, 1994) agreement more flexible, so that the management of patents would not conflict with the production and circulation of less expensive generic medications, considered essential to public health. Brazil, India, and Thailand led a group of about sixty countries in which Africa was heavily represented. They worked for access to generics, and were backed by several hundred national and international organizations, including Oxfam and MSF. For some countries with limited legal and pharmaceutical expertise, the alliance with advocacy organizations meant the possibility of receiving technical assistance. The organizations linked their technical assistance with lobbying for their political proposals. Countries concerned with defending intellectual property rights (the United States, Japan, and countries in the European Union, in particular) wavered between

11   G8 communiqué, Okinawa, Japan, July 2000; www.g8.utoronto.ca/
summit/2000okinawa/finalcom.htm.

strengthening and softening the rules. They feared that by rejecting an agreement authorizing production and circulation of generic drugs, they would spark reactions jeopardizing the entire newly created TRIPS agreement. A few months before the Doha Conference, and in view of the Pretoria trial,[12] US Trade Representative Robert B. Zoellick tried to get the pharmaceutical firms to see reason: "If they don't get ahead of this issue, the hostility that generates could put at risk the whole intellectual property rights system" (Blustein, 2001). Not all manufacturers were on the defensive, however. Indian companies producing generics were poised to take over the large market expected to result from the change in WTO policy. At Doha, the Ministerial Conference affirmed the sovereign right of nations to take measures to protect public health. Among other things, the Doha Declaration made it possible for a country to manufacture drugs without the patent holder's consent (compulsory licensing), providing royalties were paid ('t Hoen, 2009). It authorized importation from a country where prices are lower (parallel imports) without the manufacturer's or patent holder's permission. It was another two years before the issue of parallel imports of generic drugs under compulsory license was addressed, on August 30, 2003, in Geneva, with the establishment of fairly restrictive procedures. Despite the limits of the measures adopted, and the pressures exerted to curtail their application, the competition created by the arrival of generics on the market brought a radical drop in prices, which fell 99% between 1999 and 2007.

The organizations advocating universal access to antiretroviral drugs timidly began prescribing them. By November 2001, 650 patients were receiving antiretroviral drugs in all MSF projects combined. The evolution from prevention to treatment met with

---

12   In 1998 a coalition of about forty pharmaceutical firms filed suit in South Africa to try to prevent the application of a South African law, passed by Parliament in 1997, allowing the production of generic drugs. The cases were abandoned in 2001 under pressure from public opinion.

so much internal resistance that, in November 2002, the MSF International Council adopted a resolution prohibiting AIDS projects that were limited to prevention and did not include the use of antiretroviral drugs. Due to caution, treatment protocols were so restrictive they drastically limited the number of patients treated. MSF then relied on the experience of other prescribers (the Burundian *Association Nationale de Soutien aux Séropositifs et Sidéens*, and Paul Farmer's teams in Haiti) to increase rapidly the number of patients treated. From 2003 to 2004, MSF doubled the number of patients receiving antiretroviral drugs in its projects, from five thousand to eleven thousand.

In June 2001 a special session of the UN General Assembly recommended the creation of an international fund to finance the fight against the AIDS pandemic. The Global Fund to Fight AIDS, Tuberculosis and Malaria was created in 2002, awarding its initial funding to thirty-six countries. That same year, the WHO added antiretroviral drugs to its list of essential medicines. The "3 by 5 Initiative" (three million patients on antiretroviral drugs by 2005), launched in 2003 by the WHO and UNAIDS, was a major step toward providing access to AIDS treatment. Though pleased by these developments, MSF voiced some reservations regarding the absence of what it considered essential recommendations. Many in the organization believed that the use of generic drugs was not being promoted, despite the fact that generics would allow many more patients to be kept alive for the same amount of money. Some members also pushed for generics containing several drugs in one tablet, which simplified the treatment regimen for the patient, thus ensuring better treatment adherence and efficacy. MSF was also critical of the fact that the "3 by 5 Initiative" did not advocate either free treatment for patients or the right for nurses to prescribe drugs, when the limited number of practicing doctors made it impossible to treat several million patients.

In 2003, the US President's Emergency Plan for AIDS Relief (PEPFAR) was launched. The plan included the dispensing of antiretroviral drugs, which the US administration had, until recently, considered impracticable in Africa. In an article in the *Boston Globe* on June 7, 2001, Andrew Natsios, administrator of the United States Agency for International Development (USAID), was quoted as saying that "many Africans don't know what Western time is. You have to take these [AIDS] drugs a certain number of hours each day, or they don't work. Many people in Africa have never seen a clock or a watch their entire lives." Scientific arguments were needed to make the case, so Epicentre created a database (FUCHIA) of all patients treated by MSF for HIV infection. Beside their usefulness in guiding actions, the analyses produced from the database have enabled MSF to publish in scientific journals, thus legitimizing its contribution to the public debate. The international mobilization and the publication of early results on survival rates among African patients on antiretroviral drugs[13] dismissed the Bush administration's initial reluctance (Kasper et al., 2003; Ferradini et al., 2006). At a meeting with MSF representatives, Randall L. Tobias, coordinator for the president's AIDS initiative, maintained that the results obtained by several teams, including MSF's, made inclusion of antiretroviral funding inevitable in the president's plan.[14]

The number of people receiving antiretroviral treatment in low- and middle-income countries increased from three hundred thousand in 2002 to three million in 2007. Yet only a third of patients needing treatment were receiving it in 2007. That same year, 2.5 million people were newly infected, and more than two million died of AIDS. The specific needs of children—in terms of both prevention and treatment—are still only poorly covered. The treatment available today is complicated, has severe

13   The early results were made public during an oral presentation at the International AIDS Conference in Barcelona (summer 2002).

14   Report from the January 7, 2004, meeting with Randall L. Tobias, MSF archives.

side effects, and must be taken for life. In addition, the data on the efficacy of national treatment programs is fragmentary. Globally, 18% of treatment sites that provided information have experienced at least one inventory shortage of antiretroviral drugs (WHO, UNAIDS, UNICEF, 2007, p. 4). The lab test that helps assess treatment adherence and efficacy is rarely available for individual monitoring. A few epidemiological surveys make up, in part, for the lack of information on the success rates of treatment programs in precarious settings.

Today, due to their toxicity and limited efficacy, the antiretroviral combinations in use in middle- and low-income countries are no longer prescribed in high-income countries. The flexibility in intellectual property rules that made a first-generation treatment possible in resource-limited countries in no way guarantees that these countries will get new drugs, the need for which is already being felt. Nor is there any guarantee that the funding available for fighting AIDS will continue. Therefore, roughly twenty years after discussions began, voices are once again being raised, both within MSF and elsewhere, urging innovation rather than resignation.

Bibliography

Blustein, P. 2001. "Getting Out in Front on Trade: New U.S. Representative Adds 'Values' to His Globalization Plan." *The Washington Post*, March 13.

Boulet, P., G. Velasquez. 1999. *Globalisation and access to drugs. Perspectives on the WTO TRIPS agreement.* Geneva: World Health Organization.

Campaign for Access to Essential Medicines, Médecins Sans Frontières (MSF). 2001. *Accessing ARVs: untangling the web of price reductions for developing countries*. Geneva: Campaign for Access to Essential Medicines, Médecins Sans Frontières.

Campaign for Access to Essential Medicines, Médecins Sans Frontières. 2008. *Untangling the Web of Antiretroviral Price Reductions*, 11th edition. Geneva: Campaign for Access to Essential Medicines, Médecins Sans Frontières.

Ferradini, L., A. Jeannin, L. Pinoges, J. Izopet, D. Odhiambo, L. Mankhambo, G. Karungi, E. Szumilin, S. Balandine, G. Fedida, M.P Carrieri, B. Spire, N. Ford, J.M. Tassie, P.J. Guerin, C. Brasher. 2006. "Scaling up of highly active antiretroviral therapy in a rural district of Malawi: an effectiveness assessment." *The Lancet*. 367(9519): 1335–1342.

Grmek, M., R. Maulitz (Translator), J. Duffin (Translator). 1990. *History of AIDS: Emergence and Origin of a Modern Pandemic*. Princeton: Princeton University Press.

Kasper, T., D. Coetzee, F. Louis, A. Boulle, K. Hilderbrand. 2003. "Demystifying antiretroviral therapy in resource-poor settings," *Essential Drugs Monitor* 32: 20–21.

Médecins Sans Frontières. 2008. *Maputo statement. A renewed vision for MSF on HIV/AIDS from the field*. Maputo, Mozambique.

World Health Organizations (WHO), Joint United Nations Programme on HIV/AIDS (UNAIDS), United Nations Children's Fund (UNICEF). 2007. *Towards universal access: scaling up priority HIV/AIDS interventions in the health sector."* Geneva: World Health Organization.

Perez-Casas, C. 2000. *HIV/AIDS Medicines Pricing Report, Setting objectives: is there a political will?* Geneva: Médecins Sans Frontières.

't Hoen, E. F. M. 2009. *The Global Politics of Pharmaceutical Monopoly Power. Drug patents, access, innovation and the application of the WTO Doha Declaration on TRIPS and Public Health*. Diemen, The Netherlands: AMB.

Chapter 10

Contributions by Médecins Sans Frontières to Changes in Transnational Medicine

Nicolas Dodier

The periodic creation of frameworks designed to organize medicine in ways that cross national boundaries has long been observed, particularly in relation to efforts to combat epidemics (Biraben, 1976). Since the twentieth century, however, these frameworks have increased significantly and become more stable. Transnational medicine expresses the now long-term and established nature of these frameworks, which go beyond the occasional international mobilizations that can occur in response to a particular crisis situation (Delvecchio Good, 1995). Several factors have contributed to the emergence and development of transnational medicine: the rise and subsequent fall of colonial medicine (McLeod & Lewis, 1988; Van Dormael, 1997); the activities of international agencies, such as the World Health Organization (WHO), and various private foundations (such as the Rockefeller Foundation) (Löwy, 2001); and the gradual development of evidence-based medicine at an international level, based on the dissemination of a reference standard for treatment testing and approval (Dodier, 2005). The emergence of humanitarian medicine promoted by non-governmental organizations has played a significant role in the recent changes in transnational medicine in many ways. On the one hand, NGOs (and MSF in particular) have carried out a significant amount of critical evaluation designed to further the development of this kind of medicine. On the other, they have opted to fit into pre-existing frameworks to use the tools they provide, or to have their voices heard. These two aspects now need to be brought together.

Research on humanitarian medicine has so far yielded relatively little information. As far as MSF is concerned, attention has been focused on other issues. Many studies have examined the more overtly political aspect of the work carried out by the organization, which aims to define the place of humanitarian action in armed conflicts. The past thirty years have seen a whole series of debates, with which MSF has been very directly associated, proving the great difficulties involved in reaching a clear conclusion on the status of humanitarian NGOs in armed conflicts (Fox, 1995; Vallaeys, 2004; Fassin, 2006). Other studies have questioned the kind of militantism developed by members of MSF, particularly in a context of fundamental changes in collective forms of mobilization (Dauvin & Siméant, 2002; Siméant, 2001). Little attention has been paid[1] to the specifically medical aspect of MSF and the organization's contribution, in this respect, to potential new developments. Publications produced individually or collectively by members of MSF only occasionally question the kind of medicine practiced by the organization, and the place it occupies in transnational medicine.[2]

The contributions included in this publication have come at the right time. Based on examples of medical innovations produced by MSF, they provide an opportunity to approach the question from a dynamic point of view. How and to what extent has an organization that claims to represent humanitarian medicine turned the desire for change into a tangible reality within transnational medicine? In what ways has the

---

1   Except for recent research by Peter Redfield (2008a, 2008b).

2   The compilation of articles by Rony Brauman (2000) is, to my knowledge, in terms of publications, the most ambitious attempt.

organization itself been changed? In this chapter, I intend to follow some of the lines of this collective history by referring to the contributions in this publication and putting them in perspective with other publications about MSF, in order to gain a better understanding of where each example of innovation described here fits into an overall dynamic.[3]

The history of the organization can be divided into four major sequences, which in turn represent four major periods of innovation for MSF. For each of these sequences, I will show what factors drove the change (what members of MSF used as a basis for identifying failings in transnational medicine and outlining possible improvements) and the targets of the change (what they were committed to changing). By focusing on the connections between these sequences over a period of forty years, I aim to show both MSF's contributions to changes in transnational medicine and the shifts in the organization itself in its approach to innovation.

"Ordinary Doctors" Without Borders

The creation of MSF in 1971 in itself showed a clear determination to innovate in transnational medicine—particularly, in the early days, in relation to the systems in place within the Red Cross, which at the time organized a significant proportion of international assistance in response to armed conflicts. The process involved three main tasks.

The first was to change the rules for emergency workers so they could have their voices heard. The episode is well known and the story has been told many times, attracting many comments, some of which have become part of the founding mythology of the group, but it is worth retelling it here to understand the foundations it laid for future innovations. It all began

---

3   This chapter therefore needs to be read from an exploratory point of view, and not as the result of research.

when doctors were sent by the Red Cross to help people in the Biafra conflict (1967). The scale of the suffering was such that the doctors found it intolerable to maintain the principle of neutrality, which normally governed the relationship between the Red Cross and the various stakeholders involved, by remaining silent about who was responsible. They spoke in public, both on television and in the press. Their transgression was striking because it combined the roles of two different figures as witness. On the one hand, it was based on the figure of the "moral spectator" as it has been construed since the eighteenth century, which urges someone who has witnessed suffering to alert public opinion. This figure came back to the fore in the 1960s, through the new possibilities (and formats) for remote reporting thanks to new media, particularly television (Boltanski, 1993). On the other hand, media reporting also relied on the figure of the doctor, as someone who had both specialist knowledge, which was supposed to ensure objectivity, and embraced professional ethics (i.e., was sworn to protect the health and life of patients), particularly in the face of authority. The future founders of MSF stood out because they were at the crossroads where these two figures—the doctor and the moral spectator—met. They thus gave the ordinary moral spectator the tools and legitimacy of the doctor, and reinterpreted the professional defense of their patients as a duty to alert public opinion, reporting on their fate in the role of moral spectator.[4]

The next task was to think of humanitarian assistance in medical terms. In the late 1960s, non-governmental humanitarian organizations were not primarily medical: medicine just served their main objective, which was humanitarian intervention. They therefore used doctors on an ad hoc basis and in

---

4   The link between these two scenarios is not uncommon in medicine. One example from recent years is the small groups of company medical officers who are heavily involved in regular reporting on the suffering of staff working in companies (Dodier, 1993). The originality of MSF is that it has carried both scenarios onto the international stage and made them the group's *raison d'être*.

limited numbers compared with other volunteers. MSF's view of itself, however, was as an organization run by doctors and designed to assist people first and foremost on a medical basis. Although MSF's primary focus from the outset was intervening in crisis situations, the doctors it recruited were not specialists in emergency medicine. They were doctors who provided healthcare in other countries to people in urgent need of intervention as the result of a crisis situation.

Finally, MSF took on the task of reassessing the scope and range of sovereign powers in situations of humanitarian crisis, in particular vis-à-vis the caution with which the existing international agencies usually tackled such issues. They felt that it was legitimate not only to report on such situations, but also to care for people without feeling that they were constrained by national agreements. MSF sought to establish an unconditional and legitimate right for doctors to go out and find their patients wherever there was an urgent need (Fox, 1995). There were obviously negotiations with the countries concerned, but MSF believed, as part of its reassessment of sovereign powers, that it was entitled to enter these countries—much more so than the Red Cross—and make a point of doing so if deemed necessary. In certain circumstances, clandestine operations were undertaken.[5]

A Reaction to Amateurism: Kits and an Epidemiological Statistics Center

In this first phase, innovation lay not so much in products, equipment, or rules as in promoting the profile of someone who had appropriated a specific kind of knowledge and set of ethics: ordinary doctors determined to intervene in other countries when a crisis situation arose, and ready to criticize what was taking place—in the media, if necessary. The organization

---

5   One such example is the missions in Afghanistan in the early 1980s, after the Soviet invasion.

struggled at the beginning and reports highlight a glaring problem of a lack of resources in disaster areas. Doctors acknowledged that they were overwhelmed by the scale of the catastrophes with which they had to deal. Archive footage showing an interview in the field with a young doctor sent on a mission by MSF to help people hit by Hurricane Fifi in Honduras in 1974, and reused in a film directed by Patrick Benquet and Anne Vallaeys (*L'aventure MSF*, 2006) proves this point. The success of the advertising campaigns of the 1970s and 1980s marked a turning point. Resources began to arrive, including both people and equipment. The questions these "ordinary doctors" had to face began to change. The issue was no longer the scarcity of resources, but the kind of resources available: it meant defining and developing the necessary skills, and identifying and organizing the various stages of the assistance process. MSF was confronted with the problem of its own amateurism.

Criticism of its amateurism took several forms. First of all, there was a growing awareness of their own amateurism amongst doctors sent on missions. Certainly doctors who were sent out on missions had no hesitation in highlighting in their reports their understanding of the reality in the field and their ability to innovate by improvising with what they had available—and this would be a constant, both for MSF and for all those who saw themselves as practitioners. But their accounts also lapsed into an often severe degree of self-criticism on the limited range of things they really knew how to do in light of the problems they encountered. MSF doctors then found themselves facing criticism from the outside (Baron, ch. 3)[6] or from new arrivals as they began to understand how MSF operated in practice. The paradigmatic episode was the view expressed by Jacques Pinel, a pharmacist, when he was sent to work in the Khmer refugee camps (Redfield, 2008b, p.158). Tension was finally beginning

---

6   References to studies published in this book are indicated by the name of the author, followed by the chapter.

to mount in the organization around the professionalism of its actions. It crystallized around the "Ile de Lumière" operation in 1979 (Vallaeys, 2004). A first group began to emerge, made up of people who supported a significant investment in much-needed improvements in the professionalism of MSF. This group felt that the organization's main priority should be to overcome amateurism. A second group formed around Bernard Kouchner, made up of those who were primarily focused on putting out powerful public messages and who were therefore willing to live with or even keen to maintain a degree of flexibility in how missions were organized. The first accused the second of being poorly organized, unrealistic, and not taking seriously enough the imperatives of efficient healthcare in individual missions. They criticized them for being satisfied with symbolic actions, and even of taking personal advantage of the benefits associated with media coverage of their activities. The second group, meanwhile, accused the first of wanting to tie the hands of a group of militants through bureaucratic organization, or of soulless professionalization. They prided themselves on being romantics, in the positive sense of the term (i.e., people who were ready to defend a cause and take the risk of speaking out in public whenever it became necessary). As we know, the first group was to win the day, in 1979, when a vote put Bernard Kouchner in the minority.

Tangible progress towards overcoming amateurism first came in the form of innovation at a local level, at each site. Jacques Pinel, for example, a pharmacist and as such someone with a detailed knowledge that doctors generally lack, of all the issues around the transport, packaging, storage, presentation, and availability of drugs, began to organize the site and equipment in the Khmer refugee camps.[7] MSF sought to capitalize on these innovations, starting with defining and testing new treatment

---

7   See the interviews with Dominique Angotti and Jacques Pinel in the film *L'aventure MSF*.

protocols, and then turning them into real "investments in form" (Thévenot, 1986). This work was developed and made an autonomous activity as part of the first "satellite," MSF-Logistique (Vidal and Pinel, ch. 2). MSF used this structure to develop one of the basic specialist emergency assistance tools: the kit.

A kit is a set of related items (with specific instructions for use), prepared and packaged in such a way that they can be easily transported and used in a given type of situation in varying and often unpredictable locations. The kit principle predates the existence of MSF by some time; armies have long given them to their soldiers. The Red Cross used the same principle to prepare for and provide emergency assistance, starting with the famous *Materia Medica Minimalis*, developed in 1944 following a wide-ranging survey designed to assess the essential needs of people rescued from bomb-stricken cities in Europe (Redfield, 2008b). A kit designed for use in crisis situations must be able to be stored easily in a central warehouse so that it can then be transported quickly to where assistance is being provided. MSF's work in this area has been innovative in two respects. On the one hand, as part of its efforts to overcome its own amateurism, MSF developed a whole series of new kits designed for the specific situations its staff were encountering. The innovation here was the extensive range of kits available. Some of them were to be adopted and authorized for use by other organizations, such as the Red Cross and the WHO. But there was another innovative aspect as well, namely the way that MSF kits addressed the relationship between standardization and specific uses. In general terms, any kit must comply with a high level of standardization. They are designed to be mass-produced according to strictly regulated procedures. But the designers do not see the use of kits and their future development in the same way. There are two possible scenarios. The "traditional" kit can be seen as a set package that imposes a sacrosanct set of standards on users. Adjustments are only barely tolerated.[8] The kit is a rigid concept and all examples of the same kit are identical. As P. Redfield (2008b) shows, MSF developed much more "flexible" kits. The flexible kit, unlike the traditional one, is designed to be adaptable to the way it is used. The adjustments to which standards are subjected are to some extent encouraged. Changes are even meant to be recorded, retained, and worked on further so that new versions and even new kits can be developed in turn. These are "adjustable" (based on the user's own view of the situation in the field) and "evolutive" (some adaptations may in turn result in changes to the kit).[9]

The move away from amateurism was also seen in another area: being able to produce objective reports based on statistics. Initially, MSF relied on simple factors to defend the objectivity of its reports: the clinical competence of each ordinary doctor and the common sense of the moral spectator. The limitations of this policy quickly became apparent, particularly when, in the context of sometimes harsh debates with other extremely well-resourced parties (the WHO, local health authorities, and political powers), it became necessary to be able to push the introduction of evidence further. This prompted the need to invest in statistical skills and systems, such as those designed and taught by the Centers for Disease Control and Prevention in Atlanta around the epidemiology of intervention. MSF thus became part of the movement of NGOs that were made up of professionals, and equipped themselves with resources in terms of independent expertise (particularly in relation to epidemiology) in order to be able to influence public health issues when dealing with the other parties

---

8   This is typically the status of technical items in "planned" organizations (Dodier, 1995).

9   Here MSF is clearly part of a wider movement of transforming design methods in the industry (cf. Akrich, 1993), with implications for the production of kits (Akrich, 1992). It would be useful to carry out further research to examine how work related to kits is organised within MSF.

involved, in particular dedicated institutions.[10] An examination of the policy on statistics adopted by MSF reveals two ways of approaching innovation, in the same way as with their kits. First of all, as with the kits, MSF's epidemiological statistics center was an autonomous internal unit, which was a way both of encouraging specialization in the areas concerned (and therefore strengthening the move away from amateurism) and of consolidating its independence. This led to the development of the statistics center known as Epicentre. On the one hand, as with the kits, there was evidence of seeking a balance between the contribution made by codification and the pertinence of the judgments made by practitioners on the ground. Codification serves to provide guidelines quickly, particularly in emergency situations, but a degree of trust in the local judgments made by doctors (sometimes in opposition to national or international authorities) also seems to be defended by the organization. At the same time, it frequently seeks a balance between the imperatives of codification and attention to the observations made by clinicians outside the standard formats. It all relates to what C. Vidal and J. Pinel identify as a "culture of risk" (Vidal and Pinel, ch. 2).[11]

Biomedical Research Rooted in Humanitarian Action

MSF's first major investments in biomedical research (developing testing protocols relating to treatments or diagnostic techniques) followed close on the heels of the development of its epidemiological statistics center. Its research activities have continued uninterrupted right up to the

---

10 See for example F. Chateauraynaud and D. Torny (1999). A good example would be the Commission de Recherche et d'Information Indépendante sur la Radioactivité on the risks associated with the nuclear sector.

11 See also F. Chateauraynaud and D. Torny (1999) on how public health measures try to incorporate vigilance in relation to emerging risks that cannot simply be reduced to standard risk-calculation procedures (by attempting primarily to define a place for "whistleblowers").

present day.[12] They were made possible by previous events, but also led MSF into new debates and alliances. There were three main aspects to therapeutic and diagnostic innovation over this period. First of all, innovation within MSF was driven primarily by its desire to simplify treatments by drawing on a store of existing products. This was not so much about "reusing the old," because the scale of the change required to simplify something was sometimes enormous. That said, it often involved making use of drugs that had previously been ignored, because they were of no interest to the pharmaceutical industry, at any rate in that particular market, which was not seen as sufficiently profitable.[13] The fact that products were available allowed MSF to engage in research without discovering or developing new drugs as such. The focus on innovating by simplifying or adapting treatments that already existed to some extent reflects an ethical and political stance. It is about giving the disadvantaged the opportunity to benefit from scientific progress on the basis of the principle of equality of treatment for both rich and poor. As disadvantaged people are unable, in many cases, to take advantage of the most expensive, cutting-edge treatments as they stand, humanitarian biomedical research uses high-cost developments as a basis for identifying and testing those that could be made less complex and turned into a "realistic cutting-edge treatment." It must be "cutting edge" (otherwise it would simply be a cheap version of a standard treatment), but it must also be "realistic" (otherwise it would simply be an illusion). The window of opportunity between a lack of realism and discrimination is certainly a narrow one. But it is also where one of the driving forces of humanitarian innovation can be found.

---

12   The following are mentioned in the publication in terms of biomedical research: meningitis: 1988 to 2005; malaria Artemisinin-based Combination Therapies (ACTs): 1994 in Thailand, up to 2004; meningitis vaccine 1996 in Nigeria, up to 2000; human African trypanosomiasis (sleeping sickness) 2000–2003; malnutrition, Niger 2005).

13   See, for example, among the cases covered by this publication: on malaria, research into a simple, fast diagnostic method and trials on derivatives of artemisinin (Balkan, Corty, ch. 8); another example is the revival of research into eflornithine to combat sleeping sickness (Corty, ch. 7).

The second is the exploration by MSF of so-called alternative treatments. This is not in the sense of traditional treatments, but in the sense that people judge, based on clinical observations, that they have sufficiently conclusive information to try to have such treatments approved (by the national authorities, or by international agencies like the WHO), when they have not previously been through the standard approval process, often as the result of a lack of investment or, again, in markets that offer limited potential for profitability (Baron, ch. 3; Le Pape and Defourny, ch. 4). Finally, the third driving force for biomedical innovation at MSF is the fact that the organization has to deal with specific situations on the ground as a direct result of the work it does. Refugee camps are a good example. As confined spaces with large numbers of people in one area, they offer entirely new opportunities for observation (Corty, ch. 5; Balkan and Corty, ch. 8).

The 1990s and first few years of the twenty-first century were a good time for MSF to develop humanitarian biomedical research as the result of a historic conjunction of a number of factors. The first was an internal factor, namely the opportunity to use Epicentre for treatment trials. This was a necessary investment in a context where evidence-based medicine was becoming increasingly important at a transnational level. Against this background, MSF was able to take advantage of its well-established transnational position (operating in locations all over the world, sometimes affected by the same illnesses), which gave it the opportunity to set up multi-center trials or to move from one location to another in a series of trials that could then be subjected to meta-analyses. Finally, a large number of the illnesses studied during their research had already been the subject of scientific work in the context of colonial or military medicine. Many biomedical innovations of the 1990s were based on this body of knowledge and experience. Work was done on existing products that had previously been abandoned either to develop and test new protocols or, conversely, to prove that they were of no interest, primarily by providing objective evidence of the development of resistance, thus acting as an incentive to turn over a new leaf with respect to treatments that had finally been recognized as outmoded.[14]

MSF has occupied an ambivalent position in relation to transnational evidence-based medicine (or TEBM). On the one hand, the organization has worked within the framework defined by TEBM, particularly in making use of Epicentre's research and statistics capabilities. At the same time, however, members of the organization have expressed the gap between themselves and this framework on several occasions. They have done so either by indicating the purely instrumental nature of the relationship, which for them consisted of "resigning themselves" to TEBM as a way of persuading other parties based on a standard format, and giving themselves more influence in the often polemical debates between those involved, but still being conscious of the artificial or opportunistic nature of this stance, and publicizing this in various arenas (Balkan and Corty, ch. 8; Bradol and Szumilin, ch. 9). Alternatively, they explicitly showed a marked interest in treatments that had not been approved by TEBM: treatments that were supported by clinicians and particularly by local carers, but which had not been the subject of any standard studies (Biberson, 2000, p. 81).[15]

Within TEBM, MSF's position in relation to its direct contacts (national governments, international agencies, and pharmaceutical companies) has been built around three political factors,

---

14   Some of these drugs pending approval or rejection came from the post-colonial wars, particularly the Vietnam War. See on malaria: Balkan and Corty, ch. 8.

15   A more detailed study would help to explain MSF's internal stance in relation to TEBM: are there real, long-term tensions within the organization, according to the proximity/distance of TEBM? Do the same people vary their position depending on which arena they are addressing? Is it possible to identify a trend within MSF, for example towards a closer relationship vis-à-vis TEBM, as we saw, for example, in the context of AIDS in France, including from those players who were initially opposed to it (Barbot, 2002; Dodier, 2003)?

which have structured the debate for some fifteen years.[16] The first political factor relates to the kind of objectivity valued by those involved. As we have seen, there were two opposing approaches to clinical trials for AIDS treatments in France (Dodier and Barbot, 2000). The strict approach to trials is inflexible in terms of compliance with randomized controlled trial standards. It imposes stringent constraints in the way evidence is managed before reaching a decision on the effectiveness of treatments. The "flexible" approach to trials still relies on TEBM systems but assigns value, within this framework, to the relevance of observations based on clinical competences or on knowledge of the reality in the field that cannot simply be reduced to the mechanisms of randomized controlled evaluations. Until now, MSF has largely positioned itself on the side of a flexible approach to trials both in debate and in its day-to-day practice. This is also the position that has tended to be adopted by contributors to this book, and based on their accounts it is often their starting point for judging the other players involved. It is clear that there are some important nuances within MSF in terms of the approach to trials. There are several references in this book to "internal resistance" to an overly flexible philosophy (demanding more rigorous constraints in relation to evidence) (Corty, ch. 5; Baron, ch. 3). Conversely, some contributions also raise criticisms about the excessively "strict" stance adopted by researchers (Baron, ch. 3).

Compared with MSF, other players generally support a stricter approach to trials. This is the case when laboratories get involved in comparative studies (Bradol and Le Pape, ch. 1). They are therefore considered to have a "wait and see" attitude. The WHO generally appears as a defender of a strict approach to trials, which at the same time revives the more traditional criticisms made by MSF: its "bureaucratic" nature, the fact that it "stands

---

16   For a discussion of the two political factors (the form of objectivity valued and the degree of autonomy given to patients) that have structured the controversies around AIDS treatments for twenty years, see Dodier and Barbot, 2008.

firm on its recommendations" or is "slow" to react. The position of the national authorities is more variable. They are more likely to adopt a strict position within TEBM when they are examining a proposed innovation and conversely a more lax approach, compared with TEBM standards, for the management of routine medical practices. This was the case, for example, in relation to the position on malaria adopted by the authorities in Burundi in the controversy over ACTs (Le Pape and Defourny, ch. 4). In certain cases, however, this strict official position sits alongside a certain degree of tolerance for practices and arrangements that could prove beneficial (Balkan and Corty, ch. 8, on the Thai authorities in relation to malaria treatments; idem, ch. 8, on the Kenyan authorities). This more flexible approach by national governments (and sometimes MSF's own work "on the fringe") is often necessary for MSF to be able to carry out trials on treatments whose scope is necessarily uncertain.

The second political factor concerns the emphasis placed on the diplomatic relationship between nations (and therefore the extent of national sovereignty desired) in supervising and promoting transnational biomedical research. All the contributions in this book tend to position MSF as a player that stands outside the diplomatic sphere, compared with others (such as the WHO and national governments) who are closely involved in it (on malaria in particular, see Balkan and Corty, ch. 8). For MSF, the influence exerted by diplomacy brings with it a whole series of negative consequences: less concern for the health of populations, less regard for the requirement of objectivity, more time taken to set up research projects, and a preference for silent diplomacy rather than speaking out publicly (on nutrition in Niger, see Le Pape and Defourny, ch. 4; and on malaria in Burundi, idem, ch. 4).[17] Similarly, on several occasions MSF has distanced itself from national ethics committees (more so than

---

17   On the necessity of democratizing medical research ethics, see for example Bradol and Le Pape, ch.1.

the position adopted by the WHO), within the framework of a general approach that has aimed, again since the creation of MSF, and in a way that is highlighted here, to put the scope of national sovereignty into a more relative perspective (Bradol and Le Pape, ch. 1).[18] The polarized positions of the various players around the legitimacy of diplomatic-type arguments clearly converge with the fault lines created by the different approaches to trials discussed above. A more diplomatic approach often means a "slower" approach, which at the same time goes hand-in-hand with a stricter approach to trials (d'Alessandro, ch. 6).

The third political factor that tends to oppose the various players involved in the transnational research carried out by MSF concerns the supposed capacity among resource limited countries to integrate biomedicine. MSF has a clear tendency, in various scenarios, to have more faith than other players in the ability of resource limited countries to integrate biomedicine. To reuse the terms I adopted in an analysis of the controversies surrounding therapeutic trials developed as part of the efforts to combat AIDS in resource limited countries (Dodier, 2003), MSF stands in the "rapid universalism" camp, while other parties oppose it from a position of "moderate universalism." Several contrasting aspects are involved in assessing the ability of countries in need to "adopt" biomedical products: their ability to overcome operational or economic constraints, the ability of patients or their families to comply with treatment regimes, the data available, opportunities for access to treatment, the existence of specialist staff and their ability to provide training, and the level of stock available. In addition, there is the degree of "medicalization" of problems. In the sphere described here, MSF tends to attribute problems to the absence of biomedical

---

18   It would be useful to examine to what extent it is possible for an NGO to be "adiplomatic" in negotiations designed to make biomedical research possible in the countries of the South. And conversely, to gain a better understanding of the reasons given by national and international authorities why MSF, and the authors of this book, sometimes rally quickly to criticise a kind of diplomacy that has clearly seems to have drifted.

products and to target solutions on delivering such products, compared with players who tend to "socialize" problems and who therefore attribute them to socio-economic factors and, as a result, are inclined to focus efforts in crisis resolution on development assistance. A typical case is the whole set of controversies surrounding malnutrition in Niger (Le Pape and Defourny, ch. 4). With this third political factor, we find in the various controversies reciprocal examples of rhetoric that are closely linked to the previous factors (the criticism of "slowness" in the name of "speed," for example, corresponds to the criticism of the "simplicity" of MSF in the name of taking into account the issue of "complexity" [Bradol and Le Pape, ch. 1]).

Transnational medical research has thus been clearly structured, since the late 1980s, around a small number of political factors that come up regularly in controversial issues and that play a part in differentiating the players in transnational medicine along fairly well-established fault lines. MSF has occupied a fairly consistent position in this area and thus driven, through its investments in various diseases, a fairly well-defined style of "humanitarian research" that is rooted in TEBM but approaches it from an ethical and political position that combines an approach to trials, a relationship to diplomacy, and a relationship to the ability of countries to integrate biomedicine, all of which differentiate the organization both in relation to international agencies (primarily the WHO) and local authorities, and to a lesser extent to companies (which, in practice, have a limited presence in treatment trials). Alongside the innovative work in medical research that pits players against each other despite the fact that they are all working within TEBM, there was another, more radical push towards innovation that developed in the late 1990s, which aimed to transform the fundamental rules governing the production and availability of drugs on an international level. I shall attempt to describe the role played by MSF in this most recent phase of innovation.

Changing the Rules on Drug Production and Distribution at an International Level

It is worth taking a step back and reviewing how a system emerged in the 1980s which linked public health and changes in capitalism at an international level in a new way. A number of key players began to come together at that time around the idea that the pharmaceutical industry were not interested in diseases, that people were suffering or dying as a result of their lack of interest, and that combating diseases meant developing a new legal and economic framework designed to reawaken the industry's interest in them. In the United States initially, and later in Europe, these diseases were known by the generic term "orphan diseases" and were subject to specific regulations (Huyard, 2009). A little later other players, partially inspired by this new cause, came to reclassify as "neglected diseases" a number of tropical diseases which, although they affected large numbers of people, were also ignored by pharmaceutical innovation. Concerns about the fate of these diseases and the populations affected by them increased in the 1990s as a result of the fundamental changes that occurred in capitalism in general, and the pharmaceutical industry in particular, over the course of the decade. There was alarm over the increasing power of shareholders and the ensuing risks for diseases that were not sufficiently profitable (Trouiller, 2000). The creation of the WTO in 1994, with the prospect of a consolidation of the ownership rights of pharmaceutical laboratories over drugs, and a radical reshaping of the whole economic structure of the pharmaceutical industry, also led to a great deal of comment and uncertainty amongst all those who were interested in the availability of treatments in poor countries.[19] It was in the early 1990s that the WHO began to take specific steps to organize efforts to combat neglected diseases on an international level (Dodier 2003, ch. 9).

During the 1990s MSF found itself facing sudden, sporadic

---

19   For further discussion of these questions, see Chirac, Dumoulin, and Kaddar in Brauman (2000).

stoppages in the production of drugs that pharmaceutical companies deemed to be insufficiently profitable, but without linking these cases to the general cause of "neglected" diseases as such.[20] In 1996 an MSF–Epicentre symposium began to develop the idea of neglected diseases as a cross-cutting problem (Vidal and Pinel, p. 28). Work on this cause began in 1999 with the launch by MSF of the Campaign for Access to Essential Medicines, known as the Access Campaign. At the time, the Access Campaign's proposals for action focused on changes to the international rules governing the ownership, production, and distribution of drugs. These were an important development both in terms of transnational medicine at the time and MSF's earlier areas of innovation, on three fronts.

First, because the lever for change was one that had not been used previously: international trade regulations. This was the supposed starting point for major changes in access to effective treatments for disadvantaged people. This new lever within transnational medicine went hand-in-hand with the shift in MSF's activities towards economic questions and mobilizing new skills. The Access Campaign brought together not only pharmacists, but also lawyers, and economists.

Second, because in addition to MSF's work on shifting legal mechanisms in relation to intellectual property (international regulations and action on national rights), it became involved in the whole of the production chain of generic drugs. Given the decisive stance taken in this new context by (public- or private-sector) organizations producing generics, the development of international regulations designed to control production of these quickly became a crucial issue (Bradol and Szumilin, ch. 9). MSF, however, was also determined to carry out its own checks

---

20   Aventis, for example, stopped production of eflornithine, a medication used to combat sleeping sickness, in 1995 (Redfield, 2008a). In spite of promising results, in 1996, from the first trials on quick tests for malaria in Burma, the parent company stopped production (Balkan and Corty, ch. 8).

on production conditions and the nature of quality control, and to negotiate selling prices (Bradol and Szumilin, ch. 9).

Finally, this new phase of innovation was accompanied by a significant shift in the organization's approach to producers of pharmaceutical compounds. I have noted that, as far as medical research was concerned, MSF was working on trialing treatments downstream of producers of pharmaceutical drugs. This involved MSF both lobbying the companies and leaving them to take care of production.[21] Hence, from this point on, there was a twofold relationship with the companies: the organization was both critical of them and at the same time sometimes worked in close cooperation with them. This ambivalence has tended to be further accentuated over recent years. On the one hand, criticism of the companies by MSF is now expressed in public to a much larger extent and in multiple arenas where MSF operates (Bradol and Le Pape, ch. 1). At the same time, however, MSF is more involved than previously in the upstream stages of pharmaceutical drugs through its participation in collaborative bodies bringing together international agencies, industries, and NGOs with the aim of reinvesting in the development of drugs for neglected diseases at an early stage. Thus MSF was behind the launch of the Drugs for Neglected Diseases Initiative (DNDi) (Vidal and Pinel, ch. 2; Redfield, 2008b, p.135) and acts as an intermediary with Glaxo, in the context of the development of vaccines by the International Coordinating Group (ICG) (d'Alessandro, ch. 6).

Conclusion: Four Possible Histories

When we look back over all of these various phases and the connections between them, several histories seem possible. The first is a linear progression of humanitarian innovation

---

21 See for example Corty, ch. 7, and Redfield (2008b) on MSF's repeated lobbying of Aventis to restart production of eflornithine to combat sleeping sickness.

for the last forty years, which has slowly brought MSF closer to cutting-edge medical research. In the beginning there was just an ordinary doctor. The doctor learned specialist skills, innovating in terms of logistics, and going on in a third phase to explore true biomedical research, although generally working on compounds that had already been developed. In the most recent phase, through its participation in collaborative bodies such as the DNDi or the ICG, MSF has become a quasi-developer of drugs and vaccines in conjunction with international bodies and companies. The next step would be for MSF to develop its own drugs.

The second history has just as many sequences and just as many different forms of innovation. The linearity of the previous account of MSF's history hides the degree of variety. One cannot help but be struck by the ability of this protean organization constantly to renew the fronts on which it works to introduce new developments. Each sequence of its history thus equates to a break in the drive towards innovation. Targets change, as do the foundations on which innovation is based, as does the list of players involved. The group of doctors who founded the organization had a twofold target. Mainstream medicine in the first place, with its massive shifts (a form of medicine judged, in its different segments, as commercial, bureaucratic, or dogmatic), which prompts these doctors to try to develop another kind of medicine elsewhere. Then there is the silent neutrality of the Red Cross. What, then, drives change? Basic medicine and a willingness to speak out about the suffering in this world. The result is the creation of an entirely new kind of doctor. In a second phase, basic medicine itself becomes the target. It is too "amateur." The organization begins to rely on more specialist areas of medicine (pharmacists and their understanding of packaging, the kit tradition, the epidemiology of intervention) to produce new kits designed to meet the specific requirements of the situations it encounters, and to set up the statistics center needed for independent humanitarian epidemiology. In a third sequence, the target moves again: this time it is standard, routine, "official" treatments, often approved by the WHO or national authorities and used in countries with disadvantaged populations. Investing in the methods used by TEBM becomes a way of demonstrating the limitations of these treatments and gaining approval for entirely new treatments, dealing with many controversial issues along the way. Lastly, in the most recent phase, MSF attacks the pharmaceutical firms in Western countries and their responsibility for the enormous difficulties of access to treatment faced by disadvantaged populations in resource limited countries. It can then draw on the significant reorganization, during the 1990s, of the list of players involved in the drug distribution business: the rise of a generics industry in these countries and the emergence of an alterglobalist battle against new laws on international trade. In fighting economic and legal battles, the organization contributes to the emergence of new international trade legislation, to a better deployment of the generic drugs chain (from the producer to the patient), and to the emergence of collaborative consortia structured in different ways to develop new products.

While this version of its history highlights the significant new areas of innovation MSF has tackled within transnational medicine, it has one important limitation: it does not identify what is "structural" in this series of phases. At a certain level, in fact, MSF has always approached humanitarian innovation in the same way. On to the third version of its history, then: the repetition of an underlying pattern of innovation. The same basic pattern is repeated in each sequence, and always consists of two parts. First comes *innovation within an existing framework*. At each stage, MSF will seek specialist tools which, added to an existing base, enable the development of new entities. Initially there was transnational medicine that supplanted humanitarian organizations with a limited medical focus (e.g., the Red Cross).

This was followed by humanitarian medicine with specialized logistic support and an epidemiological statistics center. Next, again building on this body of knowledge and experience, came humanitarian medicine able to carry out scientific testing of innovative treatments that were becoming increasingly important in relation to standard treatments. Finally, there was the development of an entire production chain that used generics to give the world's poorest people access to cutting-edge treatments derived from research in Western countries. But in addition to innovating *within* an existing framework, MSF always adds *a change of framework* alongside it. The organization in fact always seeks to identify the problems in an established framework. This is, in some sense, the political dimension that MSF adds to each of these stages. In the first stage, for example, MSF added something extra to the idea of the "ordinary doctor": a commitment to speaking out in public, against the notion of neutrality as instituted by the Red Cross as the dominant model for humanitarian action. In the second stage, that of producing kits, MSF added a commitment to take into account the views of practitioners who actually used the kits. MSF did not simply produce new kits, but was committed to designing a new kind of kit. It differentiated itself from the technicist view of innovation advocated by designers who believed they held the key to the truth about new items and their uses. In the third stage, in addition to discovering new treatments, MSF adopted a slightly critical stance towards evidence-based medicine and advocated a flexible approach to trials that should take into account, once again, the skills of practitioners in the face of the dogma of a stricter approach. In the final stage, innovation within an existing framework was represented by the establishment of well-equipped distribution channels for generics. Changing the framework involved mobilizing people to change intellectual property law, primarily by significantly extending the scope of the argument for exceptions for healthcare products. In this systematic approach of starting

222

with innovations within a framework and then moving on to developing the framework itself, MSF reveals a fundamentally political tendency, which should no doubt be better understood in terms of how and why it has persisted through the various historical sequences.

I would like to conclude on a fourth version of the organization's history: the changing relationship with transnational standards. Transnational medicine faces two requirements on an ongoing basis. On the one hand, it develops transnational standards designed to apply to the whole of the planet. On the other hand, it must necessarily adjust to the specific local characteristics where operations are underway. Tensions, going back and forth, compromises, and seeking balance between, on the one hand, the extreme of a radical standardization of practices, and, on the other, an openness that is endlessly reconstructed to deal with the situations encountered during the course of operations, are at the heart of all the frictions seen in transnational medicine, whatever form it takes. By taking a stance, MSF has proved it is no exception to the rule. The consequences of its medical innovations can be seen as a series of different positions on the question of standards. In the initial stage, one would be tempted to refer to *standards overwhelmed* by reality. The "ordinary doctor" has a basis of knowledge and tools but also a set of core ethics that any properly trained doctor is supposed to have. Such a basis, however, seems insignificant in light of the great barrage of people and issues faced, and the doctor struggles to find a response, particularly in a crisis situation. During stages two and three, what was dominant within MSF, whether in the use of kits or drug trials, was the search for balance: operating in line with standards that themselves incorporated a *practice-based critique of standards*, one which took note of the pertinence of clinical judgments that cannot simply be reduced to an approach based on standard procedures, and tried to find an appropriate relationship between standards and practice.

In the final stage, the emphasis was on strong standards that were legally enforceable at an international level and intended to be imposed across the world. An adjustment in the law is only envisaged at a very far remove from practices on the ground: at the level of national laws, over which legal battles are waged, and which take account of specific national characteristics on a case-by-case basis. In this instance, MSF has moved away from the concerns of practitioners to act at a more decontextualized level. There is one major element missing from this history: an anthropological criticism of standards, one which takes cultural or societal diversity as its starting point and opens up the debate on the possibilities of thinking in broad terms about the conditions under which transnational standards can be combined with the specific characteristics of each society concerned. MSF's publications are nonetheless full of reflection (and even self-criticism) on the conditions for incorporating cultural diversity in transnational medicine.[22] As a number of anthropologists and sociologists have shown (Christakis, 1992; Delvecchio Good, 1995), biomedicine is always confronted, including in its most advanced sectors in terms of cutting-edge biomedical research, with the real core of evidence-based medicine and with the necessity of thinking about its relationship with other ways of dealing with people, their bodies, and the world in which they live. Will this current blind spot in MSF's reflection on medical innovations continue in the next wave of innovation on which the organization embarks?

22　This is one of the main contributions of the book edited by Rony Brauman (2000). See in particular on this point contributions by Philippe Biberson, based on the MSF mission in Guinea between 1985 and 1990, and by Eric Goemaere, based on the mission in Chad between 1983 and 1987.

Bibliography

Akrich, M. 1992. "The De-Scription of Technical Objects." In *Shaping Technology*, W. Bijker, J. Law, editors, 205–224. Cambridge, MA: MIT Press.

Akrich, M. 1993. "Les objets techniques et leurs utilisateurs. De la conception à l'action. *Raisons pratiques* 4, "Les objets dans l'action": 35–57.

Barbot, J. 2002. *Les malades en mouvement. La médecine et la science à l'épreuve du sida*. Paris: Balland.

Biberson, P. 2000. "Le désert sanitaire." In R. Brauman, editor, *Utopies sanitaires*, 79–102. Paris: Editions Le Pommier.

Biraben, J.-N. 1976. *Les hommes et la peste en France et dans les pays européens et méditerranéens*. Paris–La Haye: Mouton.

Boltanski, L. 1993. *La souffrance à distance. Morale humanitaire, médias et politique*. Paris: Métailié.

Brauman, R., editor. 2000. *Utopies sanitaires*. Paris: Editions Le Pommier.

Chateauraynaud, F., D. Torny. 1999. *Les sombres précurseurs. Une sociologie pragmatique de l'alerte et du risque*. Paris: Éditions de l'École des hautes études en sciences sociales.

Chirac, P., J. Dumoulin, M. Kaddar. 2000. "Mondialisation et médicaments." In R. Brauman, editor, *Utopies sanitaires*, 207–226. Paris: Editions Le Pommier.

Christakis, N. 1992. "Ethics are local: engaging cross-cultural variation in the ethics for clinical research." *Social Science and Medicine* 35 (9): 1079–1091.

Dauvin, P., J. Siméant. 2002. *Le travail humanitaire: les acteurs des ONG du siège au terrain*. Paris: Presses de Sciences-Po.

Delvecchio Good, M.-J. 1995. "Cultural studies of biomedicine: an agenda for research." *Social science and medicine* 41(4): 461–473.

Dodier, N. 1993. *L'expertise médicale. Essai de sociologie sur l'exercice du jugement.* Paris: Métailié.

——. 1995. *Les hommes et les machines. La conscience collective dans les sociétés technicisées.* Paris: Métailié.

Dodier, N., J. Barbot. 2000. "Le temps des tensions épistémiques. Le développement des essais thérapeutiques dans le cadre du sida (1982–1996)." *Revue française de sociologie* XLI (1): 79–118.

Dodier, N. 2003. *Leçons politiques de l'épidémie de sida.* Paris: Éditions de l'EHESS.

——. 2005. "Transnational medicine in public arenas. Aids treatments in the South." *Culture, Medicine and Psychiatry* 29(3): 285–307.

Dodier, N., J. Barbot. 2008. "Autonomy and Objectivity as Political Operators in the Medical World: Twenty Years of Public Controversy about AIDS Treatment in France." *Science in Context*, 21 (3): 403–434.

Fassin, D. 2006. "L'humanitaire contre l'État, tout contre." *Vacarme* no. 34, January–March.

Fox, R. 1995. "Medical humanitarism and human rights: reflections on doctors without borders and doctors of the world," *Social Science and Medicine*, 14 (2): 1607–1616.

Huyard, C. 2009. "How did uncommon disorders become 'rare diseases'? History of a boundary object." *Sociology of Health & Illness* 31 (4): 463–477.

Löwy, I. 2001. *Virus, moustiques et modernité: La fièvre jaune au Brésil entre science et politique.* Paris: Éditions des Archives Contemporaines.

McLeod, R., M. Lewis, editors. 1988. *Disease, medicine and empire: Perspectives on western medicine and the experience of European expansion.* London–New York: Routledge.

Redfield, P. 2008a. "Doctors without Borders and the Moral Economy of Pharmaceuticals." In A. Bullard, editor , *Human Rights in Crisis*, 129–144. Burlington: Ashgate.

——. 2008b. "Vital Mobility and the Humanitarian Kit." In A. Lakoff, S. Collier, editors, *Biosecurity interventions. Global Health and Security in Question*, 147–171. New York: Columbia University Press.

Siméant, J. 2001. "Entrer, rester en humanitaire. Des fondateurs de Médecins sans frontières aux membres actuels des ONG médicales françaises." *Revue française de science politique* 51 (1): 47–72.

Thévenot, L. 1986. "Les investissements de forme." In L. Thévenot, editor, *Conventions économiques*, 21–71. Paris: Presses Universitaires de France (Cahiers du Centre d'Etude de l'Emploi).

Trouiller, P. 2000. "Médicaments indigents." In R. Brauman, editor, *Utopies sanitaires*, 195–206. Paris: Editions Le Pommier.

Vallaeys, A. 2004. *Médecins Sans Frontières: la biographie*. Paris: Fayard.

Van Dormael, M. 1997. "La médecine coloniale, ou la tradition exogène de la médecine moderne dans le Tiers Monde." *Studies in Health Services Organization and Policy* 1: 1–38.

Made in the USA
Lexington, KY
14 July 2011